The Complete

GINSENG

Handbook

A Practical Guide
for Energy,
Health, and Longevity

Jacques MoraMarco, O.M.D.

CB
CONTEMPORARY BOOKS

Library of Congress Cataloging-in-Publication Data

MoraMarco, Jacques.
  The complete ginseng handbook : a practical guide for energy,
health, and longevity / Jacques MoraMarco.
    p.   cm.
  Includes bibliographical references and index.
  ISBN 0-8092-2971-4
    1. Ginseng—Therapeutic use.   I. Title.
RM666.G49M67   1998
615'.32384—dc21   97-35368
                                                               CIP

To my parents, Sante and Zina

Cover photograph copyright © 1997 Steven Foster
Cover design by Monica Baziuk
Interior design by Mary Lockwood
Interior art by Anne-Marie Perks

Published by Contemporary Books
An imprint of NTC/Contemporary Publishing Company
4255 West Touhy Avenue, Lincolnwood (Chicago), Illinois 60646-1975 U.S.A.
Copyright © 1998 by Jacques MoraMarco
Printed in the United States of America
International Standard Book Number: 0-8092-2971-4
 17   16   15   14   13   12   11   10   9   8   7   6   5   4   3   2   1

Contents

Medical Note   v

Acknowledgments   vii

Introduction   1

1   Ginseng—from Herbal Medicine to Nutritional Wonder   17

2   Ginseng and Stress Reduction   41

3   Ginseng, High Energy, and Performance   69

4   Ginseng and Your Sex Life   95

5   Ginseng and Your Health   123

6   Ginseng, Aging, and Longevity   151

7   Selecting the Right Ginseng for You   177

8   The Consumer's Guide to Purchasing Ginseng   193

Bibliography   219

Index   227

Medical Note

This book is based on the knowledge and wisdom of thousands of years of ginseng usage, as well as on many well-documented modern scientific and medical studies performed over the past fifty years in a variety of medical schools, health institutes, and pharmaceutical companies around the world. In all of this research, there have emerged no significant cautions or warnings about the use of ginseng in humans.

Nevertheless, if you are uneasy about taking an herbal product, have high blood pressure, heart disease, or a chronic illness, are pregnant or nursing an infant, or are taking other medications, you should consult with your medical doctor (preferably a doctor who is familiar with herbal medicine) to alleviate your concerns and to get specific advice based on your health condition and personal needs before taking any ginseng product.

Acknowledgments

This book reflects many years of training and study. I would like to acknowledge several professionals who have instilled in me a vast knowledge of Asian medicine. My first teacher, Dr. See Han Kim, was my inspiration to pursue this field. Dr. Ni Hua Ching allowed me to spend several years of apprenticeship with him. Dr. Jean Schatz integrated Eastern and Western medicine for me.

I would like to thank all of my patients who, over the past decade of my practice, have provided me with insight into the power of ginseng in restoring good health. Their cases prompted me to study ginseng in depth.

In addition, I would like to thank the many people I met while researching and studying ginseng around the world, including Professor Zhaowen Tang, renowned Beijing scholar, and D. A. and R. A. Patel at Pharmadass, Middlesex, England. I want to thank Steven Roth, president of the New York State Ginseng Association. Furthermore, I also want to thank Dr. Meng Li at the Institute of Traditional Medical Research in Beijing, Dr. Max Lattuada at Indena Laboratories in Milan, and Marianne Pfiffner at Pharmaton in Lugano, Switzerland for providing me with many detailed scientific studies of ginseng performed in Asia and Europe.

I understand that being published is no small feat. I would like to thank my agent, Jeff Herman, for taking on my manuscript.

Finally, I would like to thank Rick Benzel, writer extraordinaire, for helping me develop this book. I would also like to thank my dear friend Dr. Bernard Gunther for his assistance in reviewing the manuscript and providing wise counsel.

Introduction

The Lord hath created medicines out of the earth: and he that is wise will not abhor them.

Apocrypha,
Ecclesiasticus 38:4–5

Are your days spent feeling fatigued, plagued by energy dips, or stressed out? Are you seeking more energy and greater productivity in your life? Are you prone to chronic physical ailments or to being anxious or depressed? If the answer is yes to any of these questions, there is a proven age-old remedy that can help you regain your natural vitality and all-around good health—the potent herb *ginseng*.

Ginseng is a natural herb, part of a family of plants that have been safely used as medicinal and nutritional aids for thousands of years. In fact, the full Latin botanical name for the most well-known species of ginseng, *Panax ginseng*, literally means "panacea," or "cure-all." This impressive title was bestowed on ginseng because it was known to provide a multitude of healthful effects for its users.

Ginseng has recently become the subject of keen interest among medical researchers and pharmaceutical companies throughout the world, as increasing amounts of scientific evidence validate an array of truly astonishing health benefits. Dozens of recent general health and nutrition books, including quite a few written by respected M.D.s, are now citing ginseng as an important natural supplement that can increase energy, reduce stress, fight a variety of diseases, and radically slow the aging process.

Unfortunately, ginseng has long been shrouded in mystery and folklore, and most Americans are hesitant, if not downright suspicious, of its validity. Instead of focusing on preventive medicine, modern Western medicine, particularly in the United States, has largely disdained ginseng and other herbal remedies, preferring to fight disease, after it occurs, with chemicals and synthetic drugs. Western medical philosophy has also largely rejected the concept of mind/body balance, upon which the use of ginseng and many other herbal supplements are based.

What then is the truth behind ginseng? Is it a meaningful supplement that you should consider taking? Does it truly do anything for your body, or is it no more effective in improving your health than a carrot, as one sarcastic critic put it? Can ginseng really add to your health, vitality, and ability to resist disease, as many studies are now reporting?

This book is devoted to answering these and many other questions. My goal is to offer you current state-of-the-art knowledge about this herb. I will describe in clear, easy-to-understand terms what the recent research shows—and what it doesn't. I will explain the specific areas in which researchers are now verifying the benefits of ginseng, while at the same time alerting you to promises that are still unproved.

Two Common Confusions

Many people are confused by what ginseng really is and how to use it. Before going any further, it is therefore important to clarify these two basic issues.

The Varieties of Ginseng

As mentioned above, ginseng is simply an herb, despite its exotic-sounding name. An herb is a plant that has a soft, fleshy stem as opposed to the woody stems of trees and shrubs. Herbs usually die back at the end of each growing season, unlike trees and shrubs. With some herbs, such as basil, thyme, and oregano, we use the leaves for food. For other herbs, such as ginger, garlic, and ginseng, the root is the valuable part.

The word *ginseng* originates from the Chinese words *jen* and *shen*. *Shen* means "root"; the root is the most useful and potent part of this plant, not the stem or leaves. *Jen* means "man," and ginseng has the unusual if not humorous property of having its root resemble a man's body. A mature ginseng root consists of a main portion that looks like a body and usually several small offshoots that look like arms and legs—or sometimes even like male genitalia. Some plants even have "facial" markings on the top portion of the root. This resemblance to the human form is one of the reasons that ginseng has often been considered an aphrodisiac in many cultures, especially in ancient China, where it was believed that a plant's appearance was an indication of what part of the body it would benefit! In other words, since ginseng looked like a male with

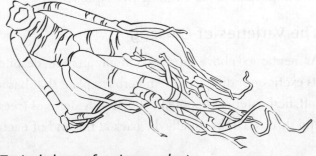

Typical shape of a ginseng plant.

a penis, some people believed that it should be used to stimulate their sexual desires.

There are actually many varieties of ginseng, all belonging to the same botanical family of plants, *Araliaceae*. Botanically speaking, a *family* of plants includes many subgroups, each called a *genus*, and each genus can include one or more *species*. The three most common varieties of ginseng and their botanical names are:

- *Asian ginseng (Panax ginseng C. A. Meyer)* — this species was first identified by the botanist C. A. Meyer in 1842, and is therefore named after him. It is usually referred to as Asian ginseng because it is found growing wild on the forested slopes of northern China (especially Manchuria), Korea, and Siberia. This is the species that was revered so highly by the ancient Chinese. Some people make a distinction within this species by asking for either "Chinese" or "Korean" ginseng, but both names actually refer to the same plant. (However, the way the Chinese and Koreans prepare ginseng differs; the Korean preparation is considered to be the more potent.)

- *American ginseng (Panax quinquefolius)* — this species is found in many parts of North America. In the 1700s and 1800s it grew wild throughout colonial America and Canada, from the Atlantic seaboard to as far west as Mississippi and Louisiana. It was particularly prolific in the Allegheny mountains, Wisconsin, Minnesota, and throughout Canada. Many Native American tribes used ginseng medicinally in the same manner as the Chinese, and its Iroquois name, *garentoquen*, was suggestive of the root's man-like appearance.

▣ *Siberian ginseng (Eleutherococcus senticosus)* — while the two species previously listed are members of the *Panax* genus, Siberian ginseng belongs to another genus, but it is still a member of the family *Araliaceae*. Siberian ginseng grows mainly in the northern areas of the former Soviet Union (but don't be confused by the fact that Asian ginseng also grows in the former Soviet Union).

For most of history, all species of ginseng grew wild in temperate forested areas, but because of overfarming that depleted the natural stores, most ginseng grown today is carefully cultivated on farms throughout China, Korea, the former Soviet Union, the United States, and Canada. Because the plant is quite sensitive, growing ginseng is quite difficult and expensive. It must be cared for very closely and protected with nets to block out direct sunlight during the day. Ginseng plants also require many years to mature, both in size and chemical properties, so the roots are not supposed to be harvested until they are at least three years old. Ideally, the roots should remain in the ground for six or seven years in order to become "medically" potent. After that time, the roots do not become significantly more developed, chemically speaking, so most commercial growers harvest all their plants within at least six years.

For the sake of simplicity, I will use the general term "ginseng" to refer to the entire family of plants, unless I need to specifically discuss one of the three main species. As you will see, there are some important differences between Asian, American, and Siberian ginseng, so if necessary I will distinguish between them.

How Ginseng Is Taken

Many people don't know how ginseng is taken, or they have an image of the plant as strictly a Chinese food or tea, so it is useful to clarify this issue.

Historically, the most common method of preparing ginseng for consumption in both Asia and colonial America was to gather the roots in the fall. The roots were then cured (dried), either in the air, in which case the root was peeled, or by steaming, in which case the root was left unpeeled. This curing process was largely to protect the roots from rot and insects so they could be stored for long periods of time. In China a dried peeled Panax root is called "white ginseng" because of its color, whereas a steamed, unpeeled Panax root is called "red ginseng" because the steaming process turns the root red. We now know that there are significant chemical differences that result from the two curing processes, and these differences affect the healthful benefits of the roots. These differences will be explained later.

Whichever drying method was used, a ginseng root was usually then sliced and boiled several times to make a brew that lasted for days and could be drunk like a tea. Sometimes the root was pulverized into a powder that could be added to water to make tea. Another common method of preparing ginseng, just as with many other types of herbs, was to soak a mashed-up root in a mixture of water and alcohol (such as vodka) to make an alcohol extract, or "tincture." Tinctures lasted longer than the cold-water brew, and were also easier to make. The tincture was then sipped straight in small amounts. Ginseng was also used in cooking; a common way to prepare ginseng was to toss slices of root into chicken or rice soup.

Today, most people do not have the time it takes to make ginseng tea or tincture, nor the knowledge needed to buy a mature and properly cured root. While you can still go to your local herbalist to buy a whole ginseng root, it is easier to obtain ginseng in capsule form, such as those manufactured by any of several reputable American, English, Swiss, Japanese, or Korean companies. The advantage of ginseng capsules is that they have been "standardized," meaning that the active ingredients from the root have been carefully "extracted" and measured so that every capsule contains the same amount of ginseng's active chemical properties.

The Safety of Taking Ginseng

You will later read in much greater detail of the benefits of taking ginseng: many people, however, automatically question the safety of it. Thinking that ginseng grows only in the Orient, people conclude that it is some type of strange or exotic herb that Americans shouldn't take. There are also those who think that ginseng is somehow related to the herb *Ephedra sinica* (also referred to under the Chinese name *ma huang* in some products) which, at the time that I was writing this book in 1996, was being highly criticized by the U.S. Food and Drug Administration because it was being dangerously abused as an ingredient in a widely marketed commercial product touted as a natural stimulant and diet aid.

The fact is ginseng is neither rare, exotic, nor particularly Oriental. As previously stated, one species of it grows in many areas of America and Canada. Ginseng is not related in any way to the plant *Ephedra sinica* and does not act on the body in the same way. Ephedra is a strong stimulant that, like caffeine, affects the central nervous system. In traditional Chinese herbal medicine it is used as a decongestant, and in modern medicine it is chemically synthesized and used in cold remedies. But just as drinking too much coffee can stimulate your body to noticeable nervousness and anxiety, the use of large amounts of ephedra in an uncontrolled manner can be dangerous. Again, however, ginseng is not even in the same family of plants as ephedra.

The safety of ginseng has never been questioned by the FDA. It has a long history of completely safe usage throughout the world; it has been consumed by literally millions of people on every continent. No illness or death has ever been linked to the use of ginseng. It is so nontoxic that the average adult would need to eat about fifty pounds of roots in one sitting to reach a lethal dosage. In short, you should have no reservations at all about adding ginseng capsules as a supplement to your diet in the ways discussed in this book. In fact, ginseng is a formally approved food supplement and is listed in official medical "pharmacopoeias" throughout Europe and the rest of the world as safe and effective for human consumption without a prescription. While most Americans are not yet familiar with it, ginseng is sold throughout the world in a variety of formulas and capsules.

If you have any concerns about taking ginseng due to any specific health problems you may have, consult a physician who is familiar with herbal medicines for reassurance and specific advice pertaining to your medical condition.

Overview of the Book

Chapter 1 provides a general introduction to ginseng and the path it has taken from a highly revered herbal medicine over thousands of years to one of the most heavily researched plants of the twentieth century. This path begins in China and extends through many parts of the world, ending in Russia, Japan, and Switzerland, where many highly qualified academic scientists, as well as major pharmaceutical companies, have been testing ginseng's restorative properties and health effects in controlled laboratory experiments on people and animals. In particular, you will learn about the most recent pharmacological research affirming that ginseng contains healthful chemicals called *ginsenosides* and *eleutherosides*. These chemicals are responsible for helping the body adapt or adjust to many potentially harmful agents, a property that has led researchers to call ginseng an "adaptogen."

Chapter 2 extends the discussion from the first chapter and focuses on the most profound adaptogenic benefit of ginseng: its ability to reduce the effects of stress on the body. This benefit is vital because, as Western science is just beginning to grasp, stress can be a significant causal factor or contributor to many physiological and mental illnesses and diseases, from depression to cancer. The stress–disease connection is complex, but there is now considerable evidence to prove that the biochemical properties of ginseng impact the body's hormonal system and reduce the level of "stress chemicals," which impede the immune system and create the conditions for disease.

Chapter 3 presents information about how ginseng has been shown to significantly enhance both mental and physical performance. A variety of studies indicate that people who take ginseng for as little as one month experience substantial improvements in their physical energy as well as greater mental productivity. Similarly, other studies have proved that ginseng greatly increases stamina, endurance, and performance among athletes. The performance-enhancing qualities of ginseng were so revered in the former Soviet Union that the Soviets gave ginseng to their cosmonauts to use in space and to their Olympic athletes as early as the 1960s.

Chapter 4 addresses the popular myth that ginseng is a "magical" aphrodisiac, or sexual enhancer. Westerners usually doubt that a foodstuff or herb can improve sexual performance, but research is now showing that the active chemical ingredients in ginseng truly have a measurably positive effect on the prostate gland and seminal vesicles in men, and possibly on estrogenic activity in women. These effects, combined with ginseng's ability to reduce stress and enhance physical endurance, make it very reasonable to conclude that the traditional myths about ginseng as an aphrodisiac have a basis in biochemistry.

Chapter 5 evaluates the long history of ginseng as a natural herbal agent that prevents many diseases, particularly heart and liver diseases, chronic fatigue syndrome, bronchitis, and diabetes. Extensive research has been conducted to test the immunological potential of ginseng. The results suggest that ginseng bolsters the immune system in many ways, especially by promoting the hormonal system, which reduces the stress chemicals that weaken the immune system. As a side benefit of ginseng, it has also been demonstrated that the herb relieves hangover symptoms and helps clear alcohol from the bloodstream. Some people have touted additional claims about the ability of ginseng to combat other illnesses, but more studies are required before we can validate such claims. This chapter will help clarify the truth behind ginseng's benefits on your health and your immune system.

Chapter 6 presents some fascinating evidence that demonstrates how ginseng can play a role in slowing the aging process and improving the quality of life for people in their middle and senior years. For example, one popular theory today is that aging is caused by "free radicals," those loose molecules that attack cell membranes and damage our RNA and DNA, causing our cells to deteriorate. Research has demonstrated that the active ingredients in ginseng spur the body's metabolism and prevent free radicals from forming. Again, the ancient belief in ginseng as a "rejuvenation tonic" appears to have a strong basis in fact.

Chapter 7 focuses on the practical matter of how you can begin to incorporate ginseng into your life. This involves selecting one of the types of ginseng— Asian, American, or Siberian—based on various factors such as your age, sex, and climatic conditions. According to traditional Chinese medicine, certain personality factors influence what type and how much ginseng you should use. These will be briefly explained for readers interested in understanding the traditional Chinese holistic view of the mind/body relationship.

Chapter 8 explains how to knowledgeably purchase commercial ginseng. There are many ginseng extract products on the market, but not all of them are the same. Their potencies (strengths) differ, as does their quality. You therefore need to learn how to distinguish a well-made product from an inferior one. You also need to be aware of how to avoid purchasing ginseng that has been contaminated with pesticides.

Turning Skeptics to Devotees

If you had never heard of ginseng or were skeptical about it before you began reading this book, you will be surprised by the evidence now existing to support its healthful benefits. As a Doctor of Oriental Medicine and a licensed acupuncturist in the State of California for the past twenty years, I have personally treated thousands of patients and have met many other people who, once they began taking ginseng, noticed positive results in their lives within a matter of weeks, if not days. I have included several of their personal stories in this book as examples of the conviction these people now have about the improvement ginseng has made in their lives. While such anecdotal reports are not scientific and don't indicate results that everyone can expect to get, I believe that you will find the stories to be an informative and inspiring complement to the scientific evidence and research studies presented. Most of the people who volunteered to let me use their stories did not mind the use of their real names, but a few were shy, so, in order to respect their privacy, I have not used their names.

◙ 1 ◙

Ginseng— from Herbal Medicine to Nutritional Wonder

Herbs and plants have long been staples of food and medicine for mankind. Nearly every civilization in the world has relied on simple herbs such as garlic, ginger, and licorice for food, and a host of unusual herbs such as raowolfia and datura for medicine.

How early civilizations discovered local herbs and learned to use them is unfortunately lost to history. Nevertheless, it is easy to imagine that most civilizations discovered edible and medicinal plants through the simple process of trial and error. Over time, each culture learned which plants and herbs were helpful and which were harmful, and passed their knowledge down through succeeding generations for continuing survival.

As an herb, ginseng is no different than many other plants that have been discovered to have useful properties for the treatment of illness and disease. Consider these other plants that have provided us with medicine for several thousand years:

- *castor beans*, the origin of castor oil, which has been used for millennia as a cathartic (digestive cleanser)

- *seaweed*, a source of iodine, which was originally discovered by the Polynesians and used as a fungicide and bactericide

- *foxglove*, from which is derived digitalis, a medication used today in the treatment of congestive heart failure

- *cinchona bark*, which has long been used to make quinine, the well-known antimalaria agent

It is estimated that there are still thousands of plants and herbs remaining undiscovered on Earth that could provide us with new forms of food and medicine. Today's researchers in chemistry, biology, pharmacology, and neurology are combing the planet for species that might unlock the secrets to better health and a longer life. Indeed, there is a resurgence of interest in natural plants and herbs, largely because more and more scientists are recognizing that the body is an amazing machine whose health is determined by extremely complex reactions at the cellular and molecular level. Today's scientists know that even the smallest traces of a vitamin or mineral can keep us healthy or save us from disease—and that, unfortunately, even the lack of the smallest amount of a vitamin or mineral can make us ill.

By Western medical standards, ginseng has gone from a "primitive" trial-and-error herbal medicine to one of the most highly researched plants of the twentieth century, subjected to microscopic analysis and thousands of double-blind controlled studies. As you will see, however, it turns out that there is actually an amazingly consistent thread running from ancient lore through today's sophisticated scientific analysis: that ginseng truly offers many healthful benefits.

Ginseng in China

China is considered the first culture to use ginseng as a medicinal herb. The Chinese discovery of the herb is likely due to the simple fact that it grew abundantly in the dry, cool forested areas throughout northern China, Korea, and Siberia as well as to the fact that Chinese culture relied on herbal medicines extensively; so they were always on the lookout for natural plants that could be used to help people.

The Chinese use of ginseng dates very far back. Some modern researchers claim that ginseng has been in continuous use in China for four thousand or even five thousand years. The first written mention of ginseng is in an early Chinese book that referenced medicinal plants and herbs, *The Classic of Materia Medica*. The book is believed to have been written by a group of Chinese doctors of the Han period between 202 B.C. and A.D. 221, based on passed-down medical wisdom from as far back as 2800 B.C. Legend also has it that Lao-tzu, the founder of Taoism, was a proponent of ginseng 2,500 years ago.

In the Chinese herbal medicine chest ginseng was not a cure for any specific disease. Instead, it was an all-purpose supplement that proactively promoted health, vitality, and longevity. Ginseng was considered a natural herbal "tonic," meaning that it nourished or "toned" the body and maintained its good health. People who took ginseng had more energy, improved digestion and circulation, and a generally healthier demeanor, and these benefits in turn led to a greater resistance to disease and hence a longer life.

According to traditional Chinese medicine, which holds that the body is full of energy systems, ginseng is said to improve *Chi* (pronounced *Chee*) — a person's "core" energy. People with good Chi possess balance and harmony throughout their bodies. Their blood flows with more energy, their lungs breathe more easily, their minds think faster, and all their bodily systems function at a peak rate. The better a person's Chi, the more harmoniously he or she lives life, and the longer he or she lives!

Ginseng is also considered to be an herb that helps balance the dual energy forces that the ancient Chinese referred to as "Yin and Yang." In Chinese culture, the body—and all nature—is divided into these two energy forces. In simple terms, Yang forces are considered to be male, expanding, and hot, while Yin forces are thought to be female, contracting, and cool. The Chinese believe that ginseng stimulates both the Yin and Yang, but primarily increases the flow of Yang energy in the body, preventing sluggishness, tiredness, and disease. When people are ill and worn down, in many cases it is because their Yang energy needs to be toned, or increased, so as to rebalance itself with the Yin component of their energy.

Ginseng is so revered in traditional Chinese medicine that it is called the "king of herbs" and the "herb of eternal life." In fact, traditional Chinese medicine has three classes of medicinal herbs. The "superior" herbs, of which ginseng was at the top, are believed to be the best because they can be used all the time; they are mild and work slowly and naturally to keep the body healthy. The "inferior" herbs of the two lower classes are the strongest and most dangerous; these are prescribed only when it is necessary to combat a specific ailment, and using them requires caution. This three-tier system is based on a fundamental tenet of traditional Chinese medicine: that doctors should proactively promote good health and prevent people from becoming ill. Giving a patient a strong, almost toxic herb after the fact is to be avoided when possible. It has even been said that Chinese doctors should be paid only when they have kept people in good health; if a patient becomes ill, the doctor has failed in his or her duty and should not be paid.

Ginseng was therefore a critical element of the Chinese diet for thousands of years, taken by healthy people to maintain their energy and resistance to disease. Even when a person became ill, ginseng would be part of a specific mixture of herbs chosen to combat the illness. Each combination of herbs was selected to treat the specific symptoms of the illness, and each herb served a purpose. Some herbs worked on the lungs, others on the kidney or heart, and still others were known to help release gas or improve digestion. For example, someone suffering from a flu that included a loss of appetite, fever, and weakness might receive a blend of licorice root, cassia bark, huang ch'i root, and spikenard root. Together these herbs would increase the appetite, cool the body from the fever, and promote better circulation and digestion. Meanwhile, ginseng would be included in the blend to support the patient's energy and vitality while the other herbs fought off the disease.

Chinese Lore and Legend

Given its importance, ginseng was a valuable commodity in China for thousands of years. In some periods of time its price was greater than the cost of gold, and only the imperial class could afford the best roots.

With ginseng so revered, a great deal of myth and ritual appeared in Chinese culture over the ages about its value, power, and use, just as we in the West have myths and rituals about grapes, wine, spirits, and alcohol. For example, ginseng roots were graded and described in rather lofty and extravagant terms, with the best roots called "heaven grade" and the lesser ones "earth grade" and "man grade." Ginseng was also associated with astrology, and was linked to the anthropomorphic constellation Orion, who could supposedly determine the potency of ginseng in each person. A famous legend recounts that in one village a man's voice could be heard calling out at night. When the villagers finally tried to find the source of the voice on the outskirts of the village, they found a remarkable ginseng plant whose root was in the perfect shape of a man. They believed that it was this root that had been calling out at night.

The most common myth that developed around ginseng was its reputation as an aphrodisiac. As mentioned in the Introduction, the shape of the plant led many people to believe that ginseng made men significantly more virile and sexually potent. High-quality ginseng roots were highly prized among aristocrats who had concubines to satisfy. One story reports that a hard put Chinese emperor paid his fortune for a particularly well-endowed root. Many men wore a ginseng root around the neck as an amulet or sucked on a root before intercourse.

Such legends and lore about ginseng spread everywhere it was used. To this day, many people still think of ginseng purely as a "magical" aphrodisiac, without recognizing that its true origins were as a general herbal medicine to promote vitality and good health for *all* parts of the body.

Ginseng in Other Parts of the World

Many people are surprised to learn that ginseng has had a very broad base of use outside of China. While the Panax genus does not grow in India, several other ginseng species were key ingredients in ancient Ayurvedic herbal remedies. The entire philosophy of traditional Chinese medicine was very influential in Vietnam, Korea, and Japan, where herbal medicines and the concepts of bodily energy systems were widely accepted. All of these cultures relied on Panax ginseng and related species in the same way that it was used in China: as a general restorative and tonic for the healthy, and as a supportive cure-all for those taking other herbs when ill.

Over the centuries ginseng's reputation also spread to the West. It was introduced into Europe in the early 1700s by a French Jesuit priest, Father Jarteux, who had spent time as a missionary in China, where he had personally seen its benefits. Due to the expense of importing it, it was mostly only European royalty who could afford to use it, and there are reports that it also became popular with several popes, who took it for its longevity benefits.

Father Jarteux's report about ginseng reached Canada in the early 1700s, inspiring another Jesuit priest to search for and find the American ginseng plant, *Panax quinquefolius*, which grew wild throughout the Canadian woods. Ironically, this species of ginseng had already been discovered by many Native American tribes living throughout America and Canada, and they were using it to relieve aches and pains, and as an energy stimulant and general tonic. While the Native American reverence for ginseng was not as strong as the Chinese, it was still a primary ingredient in many herbal medicines among the Chippewa, Algonquin, and Cherokee tribes across Canada and the United States.

The abundance of wild American ginseng seemed like a gold mine for colonial settlers. By 1720 Canada was exporting shiploads of ginseng to Canton to satisfy the insatiable Chinese demand. Unfortunately, by 1760 the Canadians had greedily overharvested their natural supply of wild ginseng, opening the door for entrepreneurial Americans throughout northern New England and the Allegheny Mountains to take over the vast export trade. By 1800, as immigrants to America spread west, ginseng became one of the top export crops across the entire Atlantic seaboard, as far south as Georgia and as far west as Wisconsin. It is said that in some regions entire villages would go out into the forest and dig for what they called "seng." Reportedly, even Daniel Boone traded in ginseng.

American ginseng was more than an export crop, however. It also became a popular herbal medicine in its own right in the American Wild West, mostly because settlers learned to use it medicinally from the local Indian tribes. In the eastern colonies too, many European-trained doctors began prescribing ginseng and other herbs to supplement their own rudimentary pharmaceuticals. In fact, ginseng was included on the official American list of pharmaceuticals from 1842 until 1882.

East Meets West

Unfortunately, ginseng's rising popularity in North America began to wane during the mid-to-late-1800s for two reasons. First, many charlatans began traveling the western frontier selling ginseng and other herbal tonics, falsely touting them as miracle medicines and potent sexual aphrodisiacs. Naturally, after enough people had paid their hard-earned money and failed to get the promised results, the public reacted bitterly to this medical quackery and slowly rejected the entire concept of ginseng as a healthful herbal supplement. The American tradition of using ginseng and other herbal medicines had simply been too brief, compared to the thousands of years of proven usage in China, to save ginseng's tarnished reputation.

The second reason ginseng lost its popularity in America was perhaps more unfortunate: it came face-to-face with the growing legions of *allopathic* doctors who were taking over American medicine and knocking aside any competing medical philosophy. Allopathic doctors disparaged all medical theories that differed from their own, including herbal medicine, chiropractic, homeopathy, and osteopathy. Between 1847 (when the American Medical Association was formed) and the 1920s, nearly every alternative philosophy of medicine was effectively banned from being taught in medical schools because it did not conform to the allopathic view of good health and disease. Conventionally trained doctors were required to see disease as the product of *external* forces, such as a virus or bacterial infection, rather than as a result of an *internal* deficiency or disharmony within the body, which many alternative medical philosophies espoused in one form or another. During the first half of the twentieth century, the premise that ginseng or any other herbal supplement might help the body resist disease by restoring vitality from within was just not possible in the allopathic view. The concept of preventive medicine, of achieving general good health through nutrition, exercise, and dietary balance, took a backseat in medicine until just a few decades ago.

The Rediscovery of Ginseng

Despite the increasing medical disdain for herbs and natural remedies throughout the West, a renewed interest in ginseng was ignited in the late 1940s and early 1950s, chiefly as a result of research conducted in the former Soviet Union. Some reports tie the Soviet curiosity about ginseng to their occupation of North Korea, where they learned that it was taken regularly by Korean soldiers. Soviet commanders sent wild ginseng home for study, and it quickly became the subject of serious scientific experimentation.

The first scientific studies of ginseng were conducted by Itskovity I. Brekhman, a medical doctor at the Institute of Physiology and Pharmacology in Vladivostok, Russia. Brekhman decided to investigate ginseng based on experiments begun by his teacher, Professor N. V. Lazarev, who was trying to identify substances that could proactively help people maintain good health and resist disease at all times. Lazarev called these substances "adaptogens," because they help the body adapt or adjust to stressful conditions.

Lazarev specifically defined three criteria that adaptogens have to fulfill:

1. They have to be *innocuous*, i.e., cause minimal disruption in the physiological functions of an organism.

2. They have to be *nonspecific* in action, meaning that they must increase resistance to a wide variety of physical, chemical, and biochemical factors.

3. They have to cause a *normalizing* action that brings the body back into balance

Lazarev had tested various chemicals without success. It is not known exactly what prompted Brekhman to think of ginseng, but he began to conduct experiments with the Asian variety Panax ginseng to see if it fit the criteria Lazarev had proposed.

One experiment in particular convinced Brekhman that ginseng had powerful adaptogenic properties. In this test, he gave fifty men a liquid dose of ginseng root, while another fifty men were given a placebo (i.e., a substance containing nothing, but which is disguised to look exactly like the substance being tested so that the subjects cannot tell the difference). All one hundred men then ran a 3,000-meter race, and those who had taken the ginseng came in an average of fifty-three seconds earlier than the control group. This astonishing difference in speed impressed Brekhman, so he began to conduct hundreds of other tests on ginseng. All these tests equally confirmed an increased performance from those who had taken ginseng versus those who had taken only a placebo.

In the early 1950s, Brekhman extended his study of ginseng to the related ginseng species, *Eleutherococcus senticosus* (Siberian ginseng). Panax ginseng was in short supply in the Soviet Union, but Siberian ginseng grew abundantly throughout Siberia. He found that Siberian ginseng had almost all of the same healthful qualities as Panax ginseng, with only minor differences.

For the next forty years, Brekhman and other Soviet scientists studied the pharmacology and biochemistry of Siberian ginseng in great detail, conducting over one thousand experiments on it, all of which continued to confirm many beneficial effects. The results were so positive that the Soviets began commercial production of Siberian ginseng extract and made it available to the Soviet public. It was prescribed for Soviet cosmonauts, who at the time were outpacing the United States in the "space race," and for Soviet Olympic athletes, whose subsequent significant performance improvements were attributed to the root. The Russians also used Siberian ginseng to help miners, factory workers, mountain rescuers, divers, and many others involved in physically or mentally demanding work.

Brekhman continued to study ginseng for many years, and became one of the most prolific researchers and writers on the subject. His work has now spread throughout the world, and his tests have been replicated at many universities, including the University of California at Los Angeles, the University of Illinois, and the University of Minnesota. The Soviet research has led a number of Japanese and European pharmaceutical companies to become interested in testing ginseng under controlled conditions and in expanding the testing to address a larger range of health issues.

Molecular Proof of Ginseng's Adaptogenic Properties

What then has the past forty-five years of scientific experimentation proved? First and foremost, the ability to chemically analyze a substance in great detail has pinpointed what ancient Oriental wisdom discovered through experience: that the extract of ginseng contains active ingredients that have measurable pharmacological and metabolic effects on many parts of the body, including the central nervous system, the hormonal system, the digestive system, and the circulatory system.

The active ingredients in ginseng are called *saponins*, which are large sugar-like compounds contained in many species of plants. In their raw form, saponins foam when added to water and are bitter to the taste. The saponins in Asian and American ginseng are referred to as *ginsenosides*, and the saponins found in Siberian ginseng are called *eleutherosides*. There are subtle chemical differences in the molecular structure of the saponins in the various species of ginseng, which is why each type of ginseng—American, Asian, or Siberian—acts noticeably differently in its effects on the body.

For example, the ginsenosides in both the Asian and American species of ginseng are broken down into two main groups, which scientists commonly refer to as *Rb1* and *Rg1*. In general, the Rb1 group of saponins is said to have the following pharmacological effects on the body:

- Depresses the central nervous system

- Reduces blood pressure

- Acts as an antistress agent

- Acts as an antipsychotic

- Enhances a weak anti-inflammatory response

- Reduces fever (antipyretic)

- Facilitates small-intestine motility

- Increases synthesis of cholesterol in liver

In contrast, the Rg1 group of saponins is said to have these pharmacological effects:

- Slightly stimulates central nervous system; increases brain activity

- Raises blood pressure

- Counters fatigue

- Enhances mental acuity

- Works as an anabolic

- Stimulates DNA, protein, and lipid synthesis in bone marrow

Although both Asian and American ginseng contain ginsenosides from the Rb1 group, American gingseng has a higher percentage. On the other hand, Asian ginseng contains considerably more Rg1 components than American gingseng. This means that the ratio of Rg1 to Rb1 differs significantly between the two species. Researchers believe that this difference accounts for the more stimulating action of Asian ginseng, whereas American ginseng has a more relaxing effect.

However, what makes ginseng an adaptogen is the fact that all types of Panax ginseng contain, at least to some extent, both Rb1 and Rg1 saponins. This combination of ginsenosides is what causes ginseng to "normalize" the body regardless of what state it is in. If you are in need of energy, the compounds in the Rg1 group stimulate your nervous system; if you are overstressed, the Rb1 compounds calm your nervous system and help you relax. Similarly, ginseng can raise your red or white blood cell count if it is low, or lower it if it is high. As Dr. Daniel P. Mowrey, author of *Next Generation Herbal Medicine*, writes about the adaptogenic properties of ginseng:

> Although it might seem that the sedative and stimulant properties of ginseng are contradictory, in fact, the CNS (central nervous system) depressant action, as expressed in ginsenoside Rb1, will be most active only when one is overly irritated or tending in that direction; and the CNS stimulant property will come into play only during severe stress. Each fraction's action is mediated by the action of the other fraction.

In short, the total effect of ginseng, particularly Asian Panax, is that it helps the body adjust to whatever specific needs it has at the moment. There is thus verifiable chemistry behind the idea that ginseng is a "tonic" that constantly nourishes the body and brings it into harmony.

Although Siberian ginseng contains no ginsenosides, its eleutherosides are similar in that they are composed of a combination of chemical agents that function in much the same contradictory way as the saponins in Asian and American ginseng. In fact, most of the research on the adaptogenic properties of ginseng has been conducted using Siberian ginseng, particularly by researchers in the former Soviet Union.

In addition to the saponins ginsenoside and eleutheroside, many other compounds have been found in ginseng. One constituent consists of polysaccharides, huge sugar-like molecules that plant researchers have shown to be potent immune system stimulants. Also found in ginseng are the phenolic compounds, a large class of chemicals that includes flavonoids, the active ingredients in plants that have effects similar to aspirin, such as white willow bark.

Another compound found in ginseng plants, *betasitosterol*, helps lower blood cholesterol levels and has been shown to have antitumor effects. Ginseng also contains a large number of "trace" minerals, such as selenium and maltol. The value of these trace minerals cannot be underestimated. In fact, recent research has proved that ingesting trace elements from natural plants is much more nutritional and healthful to the body than taking synthesized pills containing the same trace elements.

At this time, the chemical differences between the various species of ginseng are not fully understood. More specific studies are needed to compare the precise pharmacological differences and metabolic effects of ginsenosides and eleutherosides. Researchers have not yet determined whether one species of ginseng is categorically more effective than another, but most of them agree with the following general descriptions:

▣ Asian ginseng is the most stimulating and restorative of the ginsengs, useful for vitality and energy.

▣ Siberian ginseng is the most adaptogenic and toning for the entire body, and is particularly effective against normal stress and as an antiaging agent.

▣ American ginseng is the most sedative and relaxing of the ginsengs, useful for people with high stress, high blood pressure, or high cholesterol.

Ultimately, which ginseng you might want to use depends on many factors: your age, sex, health, personality makeup, and specific needs, as well as the season and geographic location. You will learn more about the chemistry of ginseng and its effects on the body as you read the specific chapters on stress, performance, immunology, and aging. Chapter 7 will go into more detail about which type of ginseng may be most appropriate for you.

From Bodily Harmony to Adaptogen

It is ironic that ancient Chinese medicine and other ancient medical philosophies understood simply from experience that ginseng improved health in many ways. We now know that they were noticing the results of actual pharmacological interactions rather than purely the results of suggestive thinking (i.e., the placebo effect), as many skeptics have suggested. Whereas ancient medical knowledge could explain ginseng only in the primitive vocabulary of a "restorative" or "tonic" that "harmonized the body's energy systems," modern science has now been able to add a new level of sophisticated chemical analysis and the revolutionary medical concept that ginseng is truly an adaptogenic substance that can help the body in many ways.

The medical importance of adaptogens is just beginning to become accepted in Western medicine. American doctors have recently recognized that vigorous exercise is an adaptogen; exercise incites a cascade of healthful hormones (endorphins) that flow through the body, enhance our physical and mental performance, and reinvigorate many bodily systems. Many doctors are also now recommending a ritual that other cultures, particularly the Swedes and Finns, have long relied on — dry heat saunas followed by cold showers — to restore the body externally and internally. Like exercise, saunas are adaptogens because they cleanse the body of toxins, stimulate the circulatory system, and produce a wide range of beneficial effects. In the past twenty years, another surprising adaptogen has been discovered: laughter. The work of Dr. Norman Cousins and others has clearly demonstrated that laughing can create significant hormonal changes in the body, ultimately helping it resist disease, and in some cases curing it. Cousins himself won a battle against cancer through laughter.

As the research on adaptogens continues, researchers are developing a more precise understanding of the actual physiological effects adaptogens may have. In the current view, adaptogens are successful because they:

▣ support the adrenal glands, which are critical to how the body reacts to stress

▣ help cells eliminate toxins and by-products of cellular activity

▣ enable cells to get more energy and to utilize it more efficiently

▣ help cells recover more quickly from work

▣ strengthen the regulation of our biorhythms

As you will learn in the remainder of this book, these are precisely the bodily systems that ginseng has been proven to influence.

If you are still uneasy with the concept of adaptogens and the role of ginseng as an adaptogenic agent, this simple truth bears repeating: the body is an immensely complicated machine that we still hardly understand. It is so complex that even with the current sophisticated knowledge scientists have about our requirements for food, vitamins, minerals, and exercise, they are still far from being able to pinpoint with 100% accuracy the complex interactions that occur at the molecular level in the body that can either keep us healthy or trigger disease and aging. We do know that even the smallest changes in diet and environment can be extremely critical to good health. Just as small amounts of vitamins or minerals from green leafy vegetables, legumes, and fruits have been linked to the prevention of cancer, heart disease, and many other illnesses, the evidence is growing that the chemicals in ginseng have equally potent life-giving effects. There are no nutritional or medical reasons to consider ginseng as any less healthful than other natural foodstuffs you eat or supplements you take.

In the next chapter, you will learn about the most significant adaptogenic role of ginseng: its ability to help the body reduce its reaction to stress. As you will see, this stress connection has wide-ranging ramifications for your health.

▣ 2 ▣

Ginseng and Stress Reduction

Yet is every man his own greatest enemy, and, as it were, his own executioner.

Sir Thomas Browne (1605–1682), English physician, author

There is probably no one in America today who doesn't feel stressed at least once every few weeks—or even once every few days. Most of us typically encounter stress in our jobs from the pressures of too much work, too many meetings, and deadlines that are too drastic. We may feel stress in our personal life as well, over conflicts with business associates, friends, or even our spouse and kids. Many of us also experience extra stress from time to time from any number of random events that throw the proverbial monkey wrench into life: accidents, sickness, divorce, financial problems, or the loss of a loved one.

Needless to say, most of us would love to get rid of the stress in our lives. After all, stress makes us feel bad. It has both negative physical and psychological effects. It tightens our shoulders and neck muscles, increases our blood pressure, and often leads to headaches, stomach pains, and other ailments. Stress also seems to make us much less effective at living life happily and productively. When we are stressed, we become angry, irritable, tired, burned out, and even depressed.

In recent years, stress has become one of the most talked about health topics. There is now a high level of awareness that reducing stress is a critical factor in maintaining good health. Stress has been linked to many illnesses and diseases, from the common cold to cancer. Today even the most traditional physicians counsel their patients to be proactive in reducing stress, typically through three practices: 1) getting regular exercise; 2) eating healthy foods and consuming less coffee and alcohol; and 3) learning and practicing relaxation techniques such as meditation, Tai Chi, yoga, and visualization.

How can ginseng assist you in reducing stress in your life? Is it possible that this herbal supplement can actually influence the body to lessen stress and avoid disease? To answer these questions, we must first begin by examining a new view scientists have developed about the nature of stress. This background will help you understand the many effects that stress has on the body, as well as the stress–disease connection. Armed with that information, you will then see how ginseng can be a powerful element in a healthy stress reduction plan.

Redefining Stress

When most of us think of stress, we are usually thinking of events such as arguments, deadlines, conflicts, pressures, and worries. However, this view of stress is actually too limited. In the modern scientific view, stress is anything that causes the body to react in a manner beyond its normal state of balance, or *homeostasis*. In fact, scientists now use the term *stress* to refer to what happens inside the body rather than to what happens outside. The term *stressor* is used to describe an event that creates the stress reaction inside the body.

This important distinction stems from the work of Dr. Hans Selye, a Canadian M.D., whose research beginning in the 1930s pioneered many of the now accepted views of stress and the body. Selye discovered that the body reacts to all types of stressors in a single fundamental way. His route to making this discovery began when he noticed that many different types of diseases made people suffer from the same symptoms: loss of appetite, low energy, depression, etc., despite the specific elements of the disease. Over several decades, Selye performed a variety of experiments on animals to learn more about what happens inside the body when various external events occur. He subjected mice to injections of glandular hormones, extremes of heat and cold, noise, and many other factors, and then studied the effects that these varying stressors had on the animals.

Selye found that regardless of what type of stressor had been applied, the animals always reacted in the same manner. This brought Selye to declare what has become the central element in this new theory of stress: that stress is actually "the *nonspecific* response of the body to any demand made upon it." While each stress event may cause a specific outcome or disease to occur, the fundamental rule that Selye noticed is that an underlying nonspecific event will always occur as well—a "stress" reaction.

Selye's perceptions of stress eventually led him to a number of revolutionary conclusions that turned the field of stress research upside down. His insights include the following principles:

1. Stress is unavoidable; the sheer fact of living means that the body constantly undergoes some type of stress, even from the simple daily events in our lives.

Biologically speaking, stress includes just about anything and everything that makes the body react, *regardless of whether it is pleasant or unpleasant, positive or negative.* In this view, stress can come from literally any change that the body encounters, whether it be a change in environmental temperature, the need for physical or mental exertion, or an emotional response to a situation. This means that the body undergoes stress just as much from winning a game of chess or getting married as it does from being fired or getting into a fender bender.

2. The body is constantly adapting and adjusting to stress to maintain its homeostasis, i.e., its "normal" state. In most instances, life's stressors, such as temperature changes or emotional reactions, are minor and our bodily mechanisms can respond to them easily and without strain. In other instances, however, a stressor may be intense or long-lasting, and we can literally feel the body adapting both physiologically and psychologically. These are, of course, those moments when we sense what we usually think of as "stress," but they should be more accurately called "distress."

3. People vary greatly in how well they react to stressors; some people handle them very well, others do not. Selye attributed these differences among people to "conditioning," which includes, on one hand,

our personal genetic heritage, and on the other hand, environmental factors such as diet and drug usage. As Selye wrote, "The same stress which makes one person sick can be an invigorating experience for another." Selye long believed that the more you could control your own reaction to stressors, the better off you would be.

The Stress–Disease Connection

Over and above the discovery that the body is constantly working to overcome stressors, another important outcome of Selye's work was a new understanding that stress has a direct causal link to disease. In his studies of laboratory animals, Selye realized that stress was part of a complex and far-reaching set of biological defense mechanisms in the body, which he collectively termed the "General Adaptation Syndrome" (often abbreviated GAS). In essence, the General Adaptation Syndrome is the body's natural self-protection against stress. However, as Selye discovered, this mechanism is a sort of "Catch-22," because in fighting stress the body also creates the opportunity for disease to creep in.

According to Selye's General Adaptation model, the body goes through three distinct phases when it is challenged or stressed, regardless of whether the stressor comes from inside or outside the body. These three phases are regulated and controlled in a complex way by the brain and many body systems, particularly the endocrine system, the glands of which produce hormones. In terms of the stress reaction, the three phases can be described as follows:

Phase 1: Alarm

This phase is often referred to as the "fight or flight" phase, because when the brain senses a danger or stressor that jeopardizes its "normal" status, it prepares the body almost instantaneously with the energy needed to either *fight* the challenge or take *flight* for safety. The biological mechanics of how the brain and the body accomplish this occurs in several steps. First, the alarm reaction begins in the hypothalamus, a small region at the base of the brain. When a stressor occurs, the hypothalamus sends a signal to the pituitary gland (considered to be the master gland of the body's hormonal system) to initiate the fight or flight reaction. The pituitary gland releases a hormone called ACTH (adrenocorticotropic hormone) into the blood. ACTH travels quickly to the adrenal glands, which are small roundish glands located atop each kidney. The adrenal glands are composed of two parts: the inner portion, known as the *adrenal medulla*, and the outer portion, known as the *adrenal cortex*.

When ACTH hits the adrenal glands, the medulla, or inner portion, rapidly secretes adrenaline into the bloodstream. As you probably know from your personal life experiences, it is the rush of adrenaline that makes us feel emotionally charged and capable of enormous physical feats. People experiencing this adrenaline rush have lifted up cars to save a child caught underneath, pulled themselves from plane crashes, or beaten up opponents twice their size. The physical strength and emotional stamina to do such acts are due to the biological effects adrenaline has on the body. Adrenaline significantly raises the heart rate and blood pressure, sending blood surging throughout the body to provide it with an abundance of fuel (glucose) for the muscles and brain. The adrenaline hormone also causes the lungs to increase their respiratory rate, giving the brain, heart, and muscles more oxygen. Several other body mechanisms change during the alarm phase: the liver dumps glucose into the bloodstream to build up blood sugar levels, increasing the supply of energy; the sweat glands begin secreting, which helps draw out and eliminate toxic residues created by the cells as they rapidly use up the glucose and convert it to waste product; and the digestive system closes down to conserve energy.

Phase 2: Resistance

While the alarm phase prepares the body for "fight or flight" within a matter of minutes, the goal of the resistance phase is to continue critical biochemical reactions so that the body can withstand the stress challenge over a period of time, if need be. In essence, this phase initiates a backup system to maintain the body's state of arousal. Once again, it is the adrenal glands that produce the group of hormones that control this phase. These hormones, called glucocorticoids, are produced in the outer portion of the glands rather than in the inner portion as in Phase 1. The glucocorticoids are actually composed of several different hormones, with hydrocortisone being the dominant one. These hormones perform several actions that keep the body's state of arousal going strong. They cause the thymus gland and lymph nodes to shrink, and they inhibit the body's natural inflammatory reaction so that blood will continue to circulate throughout the body rather than going to one site. In addition, they stimulate the conversion of protein into glucose, giving the body a continuous supply of energy beyond the initial surge of the alarm phase. As a protective mechanism, these glucocorticoid hormones also make their way back to the hypothalamus and inform it to stop telling the pituitary gland to produce ACTH; this causes the adrenal glands to halt the production of more adrenaline. This is called a negative feedback loop, because the lack of ACTH from the pituitary interrupts the GAS defense mechanism. This allows the body to restore itself as needed if the fight is over.

Scientists now know that the adrenaline and corticosteroid hormones produced in these two phases of the stress response have an unhealthy effect on the body. Adrenaline can increase the level of fatty acids in the blood, which may contribute to arteriosclerosis and liver disease. Both adrenaline and corticosteroids also damage the body's immune system by preventing it from making what are called B and NK cells, which seek out and kill foreign cells in the body. In fact, research has proven that the level of B and NK cells is greatly reduced in people with high levels of corticosteroids in their bloodstream. This explains why people often become ill after a period of severe stress.

Phase 3: Exhaustion

When the body undergoes significant and long-lasting stress, it can enter into a third phase of the General Adaptation Syndrome. In this phase, if the hypothalamus has not ceased telling the pituitary gland to release ACTH, the body will continue to fight the stressor, but in so doing, it will eventually become overloaded and exhaust itself. Exhaustion results from two biochemical events. First, the adrenal glands eventually halt hormone production, causing a drop in blood sugar (hypoglycemia), which leads to a lack of energy and fuel for the body. Second, the body's cells begin to use up their supply of potassium, the lack of which causes them to begin dying. Little by little, as exhaustion increases in severity, the body's organs start to weaken and the immune system further loses its ability to fight off disease.

As the GAS model makes clear, a direct causal link between stress and disease occurs in all phases, especially in Phase 3, when intense or prolonged stress taxes the body to the extreme point of exhaustion. The more a particular stressor causes the body to reach the third phase of the adaptation syndrome, the more weakened your immune system becomes. This is why stressors that either occur repeatedly or that extend for long periods of time can be significant dangers to your body. In fact, Selye and many scientists who have followed him have now correlated prolonged or severe stress to a long list of conditions, including:

◙ angina

◙ asthma

◙ autoimmune disease

◙ cancer

◙ cardiovascular disease

◙ the common cold

◙ diabetes (adult onset—Type II)

◙ depression

◙ headaches

◙ hypertension

◙ immune suppression

◙ irritable bowel syndrome

◙ menstrual irregularities

◙ premenstrual tension syndrome

◙ rheumatoid arthritis

◙ ulcerative colitis

Selye also believed that the body's natural adaptation mechanisms provide a clue to another significant medical conundrum: why humans die. Selye believed that over long periods of time, stress ultimately causes us to deplete what he called our "bank of adaptation energy." In his view, we are all endowed with a certain reserve of natural adaptation energy which works like a savings account. This reserve is used to restore ourselves each time we experience a life stressor. Each time we encounter an event that causes us to undergo a GAS episode, our body taps into this reserve of adaptation energy, allowing us to almost return to our original homeostasis or state of balance. This mechanism is what allows us, after we've had a stressful day, to feel refreshed after a good night's sleep; it is also why we benefit from a relaxing vacation after several consecutive weeks of physically or mentally hard work. This adaptation mechanism allows us to rebuild our supplies of energy and lets our brain and glands return to their normal functioning.

The problem is, according to Selye, that for each stressful event that takes us into the third phase of exhaustion, we are left chemically scarred. Using the metaphor of the bank account, stress forces us to cash in our savings account. Over time, with each withdrawal from our account, we eventually deplete our adaptation energy. We ultimately end up in an exhausted state with no adaptation energy left to save us, and we die either from a disease, from which we can no longer protect ourselves, or from the natural death of our organs.

Selye's work on the nonspecific nature of stress and the body's adaptation defense mechanisms is now widely accepted and forms the basis for much of today's research in stress reduction and disease prevention. The two most important concepts to remember from Selye's work are that the body is constantly being taxed to adapt to stressors that may be either good or bad, and the more you experience stressors that cause the body to enter the exhaustion phase, the more at risk you are for disease or death.

The Ginseng–Stress Reduction Connection

You are probably wondering at this point how ginseng relates to Dr. Selye's research on the nature of stress and the sophisticated adaptation process of the body's natural defenses. The answer goes back to the fundamental idea that ginseng is an adaptogen that helps the body rebalance itself in the face of any condition. The active ingredients in ginseng allow the body to adjust to the demands of any stressor, whether it requires raising or lowering your blood pressure or glucose levels, or speeding up or slowing down your metabolism and hormone production. Whatever the event, ginseng helps the body respond in a more healthful manner so that it can meet the challenge without exhaustion.

There are literally hundreds of experiments that indicate that ginseng improves the body's ability to function when it is under mental or physical duress. Here are a few:

▣ *Extreme Temperatures:* The Arctic region presents a particularly harsh climatic environment, with below-zero temperatures on a daily basis. In this experiment, one thousand workers at a polar station were given ginseng for five months. Over a period of one year, there was a 40% reduction in days lost from work and a 50% reduction in general sickness compared to the previous year.

▣ *Demanding Physical Labor and Harsh Environmental Conditions:* In this study, 1,200 workers at a car factory in the former Soviet Union were given ginseng in the spring and autumn for two years. By the end of the study, the incidence of illness in this group had fallen 20% versus another group of workers who had not been given ginseng. In the same study, it was also found that while at the beginning of the study the two groups of workers had the same proportion of individuals with high blood pressure, by the end of the study the proportion was 3.5 times lower among those who had taken ginseng.

▣ *Intense Mental Work:* In this study, Russian telegraph operators were asked over two tests to quickly encode a special message. Those given a placebo increased their speed only slightly in the second test, but made 28% more mistakes than in the first test, while those operators who were given ginseng made 10% fewer mistakes in the second test. In another study, thirty-three young Swedish men had to identify a pattern of letters in a random set; those who had taken ginseng made approximately half as many errors on one test as those who had not taken ginseng, and two-thirds as many errors on a second test.

▣ *Stamina:* In a study conducted in London by noted British ginseng researcher Steven Fulder, nurses who worked at night were given ginseng under double-blind conditions, i.e., no one knew who received a placebo and not real ginseng. Those who had been given ginseng felt more capable and alert, and, when tested, had better speed and coordination.

Every human study has consistently affirmed that the use of ginseng correlates positively with higher rates of physical and mental performance, more stamina, less fatigue, and an increased resistance to disease. Many people who took ginseng in experiments have also commented on a general sense of well-being and satisfaction they achieved while using it. Such assessments are clearly subjective, but they nevertheless indicate a positive psychological attitude that people say exists for them when using ginseng.

In addition to the human studies, there have been literally thousands of experiments conducted on laboratory animals, all of which have equally confirmed the benefits of ginseng on performance and productivity. It is also important to note that such animal studies are proof that the benefits of ginseng are not related to a placebo effect, since animals obviously cannot distinguish between a placebo and the real substance being tested.

In one of the most well-known animal experiments, 120 mice were given a stamina test in which they were put in water to swim until they were exhausted. They were then taken out of the water and allowed to rest. Typically mice that had to swim a second time would become exhausted after a much shorter time than after the first test. However, when given ginseng, their second swim time nearly doubled. In other similar tests with mice that were given ginseng for four weeks, the average swimming time of these mice was 50% longer than the time of those mice that were not given ginseng. In a test with mice climbing a swinging rope, those given ginseng performed significantly better than those not given ginseng.

In tests of learning, too, rats that were given a shock stimulus after the sound of a buzzer learned to avoid the shock much more quickly when they were injected with ginseng. When the test was modified so that a buzzer was no longer followed by a shock, a larger percentage of rats who had been given ginseng unlearned the response than those not given ginseng. In another test, mice were given exercise till they were fatigued. They were then released to explore an unknown area. The mice that had been given ginseng were more willing to explore than those that had not been given ginseng. The list of tests on animals is endless, and in each case, the results consistently confirm that animals that have been given ginseng exhibit better performance, stamina, endurance, and adaptation to stress.

The Inner Workings of Ginseng

How does ginseng affect the body and improve its ability to withstand stress? It comes down to its active chemical properties, the saponins and trace elements contained in ginseng roots. Like the nutrients in any foodstuff, these saponins chemically interact with the chemical events in the body. But in the case of ginseng, the nutrients literally "moderate" the stress reaction so that the body remains stronger, healthier, and better able to handle any challenge.

Research indicates that this moderating influence occurs because ginseng directly affects the body's hormonal system. The most important evidence for this indicates that ginseng alters the functioning of the adrenal glands, which as the GAS model suggests, are the body's first line of defense against stressors. Ginseng's influence on the adrenal glands has been measured in several controlled studies in which one group of lab animals was given ginseng injections while another group of test animals was not. Both groups were then exposed to stress. The group given the ginseng showed significantly less enlargement of the adrenal glands than the group not given ginseng. Less enlargement indicates that the adrenal glands were being taxed much less; in other words, they were less stressed because of the ginseng. As a double check of such studies, another research experiment removed the adrenal glands from lab animals. The animals were then given performance tests, but without their adrenal glands their performance was significantly worse, even when given ginseng. By deduction, this indicated that ginseng worked on the adrenal glands.

Similarly, in another study, ginseng was shown to inhibit the adrenal glands from atrophying (shrinking) after severe stress.

The specific biology of how ginseng protects or supports the adrenal glands is not precisely known, but one study indicates that ginseng initially speeds up the production of hormones from the adrenal glands and then aids in quickly restoring the glands to their normal state. This effect would indicate that ginseng helps the adrenals react to stress more quickly in Phase 1 (the alarm phase) and recover from it more quickly in Phase 2 (the resistance phase). Steven Fulder writes,

> In stress, ginseng helps the adrenal glands to mount an immediate hormonal response; more stress hormones are released and more manufactured. But when stress stops, the adrenal glands shut down more quickly. If stress is long and severe, the glands conserve their resources and do not release so much hormone.

Of further interest, several studies indicate that ginseng may actually influence the triggering mechanisms "upstream" of the adrenal glands, i.e., the pituitary gland and the hypothalamus. Recall that the hypothalamus must first signal the pituitary gland to produce ACTH, which then triggers the adrenals to produce the adrenaline and corticosteroid hormones during Phases 1 and 2. The link between these three elements of the endocrine system is so strong that it is often referred to as the hypothalamus/adrenal/pituitary axis. A number of studies suggest that ginseng influences not only the adrenal glands but the entire axis, thus playing an even larger role than simply moderating the action of the adrenal glands.

Again, the precise pharmacology of this process is not yet completely understood, but experiments indicate that the active ingredients in ginseng (the ginsenosides or eleutherosides) may first affect the production of ACTH in the pituitary gland. There is a chemical in the adrenal gland that changes when ginseng is administered. However, in laboratory animals whose pituitary gland has been removed, this chemical does not change, indicating that ginseng may first affect the production of ACTH, which then directs the adrenal gland to function. Unfortunately, scientists have yet to pinpoint the interactions between the hypothalamus, the pituitary gland, and the adrenal glands, so it is still too early to say with conviction how the three parts control the stress response and where ginseng has the most critical effect.

Ginseng and Your Metabolism

There is also evidence demonstrating that ginseng plays a role in assisting several other aspects of your metabolism during periods of increased demand on the body. Stress requires the body to gather all its energy and be ready to produce more as needed. It is known that cells transfer energy from carbohydrates and other food molecules through mitochondria, small bodies within the cells that act as miniature power plants. The conversion process from food to energy requires an enzyme called ATPase, which assists in storing the energy as a compound called adenosine triphosphate (ATP). Research has shown that ginseng facilitates the functioning of this enzyme, indicating that ginseng acts as a catalyst for energy production.

The liver also plays an important role in the stress response. It stores glucose for energy, but when adrenaline is pumped into the body during the stress response, the liver dumps the glucose into the bloodstream to provide more energy for Phase 1. As the stress response continues, the liver also resynthesizes new glucose from the lactic acid produced by muscles. The resynthesis process requires protein and RNA. In this regard, ginseng has been shown to increase the production of RNA in animals, thus improving their ability to regain energy when the stress response calls for it. There are also a number of other metabolic processes (which are far too technical to be discussed in this book) with which ginseng has been positively correlated as contributing to their efficiency. Overall, there is a vast amount of evidence suggesting that ginseng helps the body produce and utilize energy, both of which are critical processes in the stress reaction.

Finally, ginseng also appears to make people feel better by having a positive chemical effect on the brain. The explanation at this time is that ginseng improves the balance among various brain chemicals such as serotonin and dopamine. Ginseng administered to rats has been shown to increase biogenic amine content in the brain, adrenals, and urine.

Toward a Unified Theory of Ginseng as an Adaptogen/Antistress Agent

The preceding information summarizes the current state of knowledge about the chemistry of ginseng and how ginseng supports the body during the stress response. Obviously, much more research remains to be undertaken toward precisely understanding the herb's biochemistry and pharmacology.

However, it is curious to note that while Dr. Selye recognized the concept that the body always has a "nonspecific" stress response, the Soviets coined the term "adaptogen" to describe plants or drugs that have "nonspecific" healthful effects. Obviously, the two concepts are parallel in principle. The logical question is, is ginseng a foodstuff or natural drug that can help the body's nonspecific stress response because it has

nonspecific effects? Can ginseng fulfill the requirements of a medicine that fits neatly into Selye's concept of assisting the body in its natural adaptation
mechanism?

Although the validity of ginseng as an adaptogen
has long been questioned, many people now believe
the answer is yes, that ginseng is perhaps one of the
most important adaptogens. Steven Fulder has even
proposed an intriguing hypothesis that helps to unify
Selye's stress concepts with the workings of ginseng
as a true adaptogen. Fulder strongly believes that
ginseng directly affects many hormonal functions
of the body, beginning with the hypothalamus. In
his view, ginseng primes all the cells of the body
for the release of the stress hormones—only if and
when the body is challenged by a stressor. Ginseng
sensitizes the hypothalamus so that it is prepared to
instruct the pituitary gland to produce ACTH more
quickly and also shut down the adrenal glands more
quickly than it otherwise would have done without
ginseng. In this view, ginseng acts as a preparatory
agent to speed up the alarm reaction in the hypothalamus so that the body can react more aggres-
sively to stress; it then acts as a moderator, shutting
down the stress hormone system more rapidly so
that the body does not reach the exhaustion phase
in which it overexerts itself and ultimately destroys
itself.

Fulder makes an intriguing observation to support his hypothesis: that there is a less-than-coincidental similarity between the chemical composition of ginseng and that of the body's stress hormones. As mentioned in Chapter 1, all varieties of ginseng are composed of many compounds, but chief among them are the saponins. As Fulder points out, the saponins in ginseng, called *triterpenoids*, are very similar in chemical structure to the steroids in the body, such as cortisone, cholesterol, estrogen, and testosterone. Could it be, Fulder wonders, that the saponins in ginseng actually reinforce or complement the steroidal hormones produced in the body during stress? This chemical similarity would explain why ginseng appears to strongly affect the hypothalamus, the production of ACTH, and the adrenals.

Since Fulder proposed his hypothesis, at least one experiment has seemed to confirm that animals given ginseng produce more steroids in the brain, thereby increasing their ability to handle stress. However, at this time more research is needed to validate the chemical similarities and to determine more precisely the actions of ginseng on the hypothalamus, pituitary, and adrenals.

Nevertheless, enough research has been done to suggest a logical fit between the concept of an adaptogen (particularly ginseng) and the body's natural adaptation mechanism. The logic is as follows:

1. The hormonal system is one of the body's first lines of defense against stress. As Selye found, the GAS always involves the hypothalamus, pituitary gland, and adrenal axis; whenever there is stress, these systems react by producing the hormones that control the stress response. In some cases, the hormonal system stimulates the body by increasing blood pressure, metabolism, and energy production. In other cases, the hormonal system slows or shuts the body down, as in sleep or relaxation. In short, the hormonal system is truly the body's primary adaptogenic system, or at least one of them.

2. Research indicates that ginseng has a strong effect on the hormonal system of the body, working closely with the adrenals and perhaps even affecting the hypothalamus, as Fulder suggests. Ginseng may also have a chemical link to the steroids in the body, complementing or reinforcing their actions.

3. The wide range of effects that ginseng has on the body and its sometimes contradictory nature may be due to the fact that ginseng complements or reinforces the hormonal system, which likewise has contradictory functions. Whether ginseng simply primes the hypothalamus or chemically reinforces the adrenal steroids is not clear, but the fact is, its adaptogenic properties can be explained by its effects on the hormonal system.

Clearly, this area is a fertile one for further exploration, but it does explain how ginseng might be an adaptogen. It also points the way to the possible existence of other adaptogens. In fact, the similarity in chemical structure between saponins and human steroids reinforces why many other plants that contain saponins, including licorice, thyme, sugar beets, and sarsaparilla, have long been considered to have significant healthful properties. It may be that there are many adaptogens that have a wealth of beneficial effects on the body if used in the right way. At the moment though, the most potent of these still appears to be ginseng.

Putting It All Together

As years of research are slowly confirming, ginseng creates specific and observable changes in the body that correlate highly with the lessening of the stress reaction. This research has many implications for anyone who is concerned about reducing or eliminating stress from his or her life. The bottom line is that taking ginseng can be an important ingredient in your stress-reduction program. In biochemical terms, ginseng helps your entire hormonal system combat stressors by supporting your adrenal glands and stimulating your body's metabolism. These chemical events in your body translate into many powerful effects: ginseng improves your physical and mental performance, increases your stamina, and prevents many acute illnesses caused by fatigue and stress.

While this chapter has defined stress in Selye's terms, as any event that disrupts the body's normal functioning, you may be wondering if ginseng will help you with the stresses that we typically encounter: deadlines, arguments in the office, family squabbles, financial problems, etc. In my view, the answer is definitely yes. Although the connection between ginseng and modern life may appear to be very indirect, stressors like office politics, congested highways, and bad service in retail stores also call for endurance, stamina, and resistance!

Ginseng and the stress–disease connection deserve special attention. Although a later chapter in this book will present many more details about the research on ginseng and its ability to spur the body's immunological system to combat specific illnesses, this chapter has demonstrated that ginseng helps the body avoid excessive and prolonged stress, thereby reducing your chances of contracting a host of stress-related diseases. For this reason, adding ginseng to your diet to support your natural antistress mechanisms is highly recommended.

Let me add one final thought to this chapter. It is obviously foolish to suggest that ginseng alone can help you eliminate or reduce the many potential negative ramifications of stress in your life. If you are seeking to lessen the amount of stress that you encounter, you need a comprehensive attack that includes good nutrition, regular exercise, and the use of relaxation techniques. Learning about each of these will prove valuable if you are serious about reducing your stress and living a healthier life.

▣3▣

Ginseng, High Energy, and Performance

Our own physical body possesses a wisdom which we who inhabit the body lack. We give it orders which make no sense.

Henry Miller
(1891–1980),
U.S. author

Your mind and body function together like a miraculous machine. Day in and day out, they accomplish the myriad tasks you give them, from writing memos and going to meetings, to reading books, playing sports, or caring for your children. Hour after hour, you are constantly tapping into your mental and physical resources. To perform even the simplest mental task, you must move energy through billions of brain cells in order to use your analytic and creative thinking skills. To perform any physical task or sport, you need to call upon your muscles to expand and contract tirelessly and in extremely complex ways for both gross and fine motor movements.

Unfortunately, for the majority of us, getting the maximum performance out of our mind and body is an elusive goal. We are only occasionally able to achieve "peak performance," in which our mind is quick and sharp at coming up with answers to our problems, or our body is able to perform effortlessly with strength and vigor whatever challenge we give it. For most of us, the level of our performance might best be classified as normal or ordinary. Whether it's a simple game of tennis, a jog through the park, or a lengthy meeting at work, we too often end up feeling tired and exhausted from the events of our days.

There are a variety of reasons for mediocre physical and mental performance. First, as mentioned in the last chapter, the many stressors we encounter in our daily life deplete our body's resources and prevent us from reaching or staying at our maximum level of output for long periods of time. Stressors wear the mind and body down, causing many types of physical and emotional problems that make it difficult for us to think clearly or stay at a physical task with constant energy and stamina. There are also the normal temptations of the good life—too much food, too many activities, and too much pressure. Such excesses invariably imbalance our mind and body, creating a negative chain reaction that cascades from one bodily system to another and ultimately prevents us from sustaining a peak level of functioning.

What steps can you take if you want to improve the quality of your mental and physical performance? Obviously, the first step is to make a commitment to living a healthier lifestyle. In general, a healthier lifestyle means a diet of more nutritious foods, eaten in smaller quantities, combined with exercise on a consistent and regular basis to strengthen your muscles and build up your endurance. Another aspect of a healthier lifestyle is the development of a positive attitude and more resiliency toward life's problems. These characteristics help you improve your mental powers and stamina so that you can use your fullest analytic and creative skills to resolve the challenges you encounter at work or at home. In fact, research has shown that people with a positive view of life tend to be far more productive in their work and significantly less prone to anxiety and depression than people who approach problems with a negative attitude.

Needless to say, there is one other ingredient that you can add to your lifestyle to boost your mental and physical performance: ginseng. In this chapter, you will learn how ginseng has been linked through hundreds of experiments to significantly increased physical strength and endurance, higher levels of productivity, better mental concentration, and faster learning.

Physical Performance

Although traditional Chinese medicine has long regarded Asian ginseng as a stimulant that energizes the body, the experiments conducted by Itskovity Brekhman were actually the first to specifically document the power of ginseng to boost physical performance. As mentioned earlier, one of Brekhman's first experiments using Asian ginseng involved one hundred men in a 3,000-meter run. To reiterate, he discovered that the group of fifty men who had taken ginseng before the race finished at an average of fifty-three seconds earlier than the control group that had taken a placebo. The clear-cut results of this study excited Brekhman and many other researchers across the globe, and led them to perform hundreds of other experiments to further test the relationship between ginseng and physical performance.

Today, more than forty years after that experiment, the general conclusion that Brekhman and every other such scientist have drawn from their research is that ginseng significantly enhances a person's physical capacities and endurance. In every case, the results have consistently shown that a regular dosage of ginseng over a period of time—usually ten to twelve weeks— lowers the heart rate during physical exertion, improves the body's lung capacity and use of oxygen, and reduces the level of lactic acid in the blood stream (which causes fatigue in the muscles).

Here is a brief synopsis of a few of the most noted experiments. Let's begin by looking at the effects of ginseng on the average person's physical capacities. In one experiment conducted at the University of Chieti in Italy, the subjects were normal, healthy males who were tested for their ability to withstand increasing amounts of physical exertion. This study involved fifty men between the ages of twenty-one to forty-seven. For six weeks half of the men were given a pill containing the ginseng extract G115 (made by a well-known European company) plus vitamins and minerals, while the other half were given a placebo. The men were then tested on a treadmill at varying speeds and steepness of incline, thereby measuring what is called *workload*. The steeper the incline, the higher the workload. An individual's ability to handle a higher workload with less exertion was an indication of better performance. Following the first set of tests, the groups were switched and the other half was given the ginseng/vitamin/mineral mixture. The men were then retested. Neither group knew which pill they were given at any time. In both phases of the experiment, the group of men that had taken the ginseng capsules had lower levels of oxygen consumption, lower heart rates, lower plasma lactate levels, and lower carbon dioxide production—all indications of an increase in the body's ability to handle the physical workload with less exertion. That the groups were switched midway indicates that the effects of the ginseng were completely uniform; i.e., they cannot be attributed to one group of men being more physically capable than the other.

It is also interesting to note that in this study twenty-three of the men had lower levels of oxygen in the blood before the start of the program, indicating that they were more or less in "worse shape" than the others. However, over the course of the six weeks during which the men took the ginseng/vitamin/mineral mixture, this group actually showed higher levels of improvement than the men who were in better shape at the start. This suggests that ginseng may be especially beneficial for people who seldom exert themselves or get little exercise.

The Italian study is not unique in demonstrating the power of ginseng to improve physical capacity. In a similar experiment done in Sweden on thirty-eight normal healthy men from a factory, all between the ages of fifty and fifty-four, very similar results were achieved over eight weeks between men who had taken a ginseng extract versus those who had taken a placebo. In this study the subjects were tested on a stationary bicycle, being subjected to increasing workloads until they reached exhaustion. The results indicated that the men who had taken ginseng had a greater workload capacity, lower heart rates, and lower lactate levels than the men who had taken a placebo. In another study of 120 male and female subjects be-

tween the ages of thirty and sixty, the participants between the ages of forty and sixty who had taken a standardized extract of ginseng for twelve weeks had
greater pulmonary function as well as an increased capacity to perform on visual and acoustic reaction tests.
And a recent study at the University of Toronto compared two groups, one which had taken American ginseng and one which had taken a placebo, for ninety
days. Those subjects who had taken ginseng were measured to have a significant reduction in ventilation,
that is, the amount of air they consumed while exer-
cising. This indicated that ginseng helped make their
breathing rate more efficient.

These are just a few of the experiments that have
been conducted on average subjects with the goal of
directly testing performance. In addition, a number of
other studies have indirectly confirmed enhanced
physical performance. For example, a Soviet experiment was conducted over two months on sailors living
in the tropics, who had to endure high temperatures
and difficult working conditions. In that study, twenty-
nine of the sailors were given ginseng and forty-eight
were given a placebo. Nearly three-quarters of the men
who had taken ginseng demonstrated increased performance, as measured by their ability to adapt to the
harsh conditions and to perform difficult mental and
physical labor. These men also had lower heart and
breathing rates, as well as decreased blood flow. The

Soviets ultimately found ginseng so effective in enhancing physical performance that they gave it to their
cosmonauts, who had to remain in space for periods
far longer than did their American counterparts. The
Soviets also undertook a program to make ginseng
widely available to factory workers, miners, truck drivers, and other hard laborers who had to endure extremely harsh working conditions in their professions.

The Athlete's Friend

One area of life where physical performance counts
greatly is athletics. For this reason, a large number of
experiments have been conducted to measure the effects of ginseng on sports performance. All of them
confirm a striking increase in many measures of performance, including strength, endurance, concentration, and focus. Here are a few of the most noted
experiments:

- In a series of experiments involving Soviet Olym-
  pians, thirty male and female athletes took ginseng
  extract before going to bed and again in the morning before their workouts. All of these athletes, who
  included sprinters, high jumpers, runners, and
  marathoners, noted higher levels of endurance in
  the performance of their sport as well as a readiness
  to train longer and harder. The control group of ath-

letes who did not take ginseng were much less active. Researchers also found that the restoration of
pulse, blood pressure, and muscle tone required less
time in the ginseng group than in the control group.

▣ In one experiment involving male German athletes,
a group of fourteen who took ginseng twice daily
had significantly higher rates of oxygen uptake and
lower serum lactate levels in their blood, compared
to a placebo group during training sessions over ten
weeks. In two similar types of sports training experiments with twenty subjects and thirty subjects re-
spectively, researchers determined that the athletes
continued to experience performance gains for
three weeks after stopping their use of ginseng.

▣ In an experiment with Soviet runners, 34 participants were given 2 ml of ginseng 30 minutes before
a race, 33 participants were given 4 ml of ginseng,
and a control group of 41 participants were given no
ginseng. The results of the 10-kilometer race corre-
sponded to the amount of ginseng given: the 4 ml
group averaged 45 minutes; the 2 ml group, 48.7
minutes; and the control group, 52.6 minutes.

▣ In a study in Switzerland, thirty athletes between
the ages of eighteen and thirty-one, who were all in
top shape and trained regularly, were given either
ginseng, ginseng plus Vitamin E, or a placebo for
nine weeks. Those who had received either the gin-

seng or ginseng plus Vitamin E had substantially higher levels of oxygen absorption and lower heart rates than the placebo group.

As noted in Chapter 2, hundreds of experiments using animals have produced performance enhancing results similar to these human studies.

The Story of American Triathlon Notable Eric Harr

For me, one of the most significant personal stories exemplifying the power of ginseng in athletics is that of Eric Harr, the American triathlete who has gained the attention of the sports world in recent years. Eric officially began his professional triathlon career in 1994 and within that first year was declared to be the "Rookie of the Year." However, in early 1995 his performance began to decline due to his strenuous training schedule and, as Eric freely admits, to his overconfidence from having been declared Rookie of the Year. Eric and his coach therefore set out to improve his progress and renew his goal to try out for the American Olympic team in 2000.

One of the first things Eric's coach did was to explore the use of ginseng. The coach had heard of ginseng and suggested that Eric begin taking it along with the other "ergogenic" dietary supplements that he takes daily to help his body reduce fat and increase its energy output. Eric explains that for a professional athlete of his caliber, the goal is to burn body fat, which is much more efficient than burning glucose. Therefore, he takes many supplements to improve his metabolism. Eric and his coach selected a ginseng product, but to be sure it would help him, they performed a "ramp test," which allowed them to isolate and quantify the specific effects the ginseng was having. Eric explained that they do this for any new supplement he decides to take because, naturally, he is not interested in taking a supplement that does not create a beneficial effect. To test a product, Eric therefore abandons all other supplements he would ordinarily take for three weeks, during which time he tries out the new supplement. Over this three-week test period, Eric does a stationary bicycle test each day with a meter attached to measure his energy output. A meter is also attached to his body to measure his heart rate. After three weeks on any new supplement, Eric discontinues taking the new substance and returns to his usual diet for three more weeks to compare results. This six-week process is then repeated to double-check the results.

In this case, he tried one capsule each of Korean and Siberian ginseng in the morning. By the end of the twelve-week period testing ginseng in this manner, Eric was astounded. He told me that in both test periods, the ginseng had increased his output by an astounding 8%, an extremely high level of improvement from a single supplement! Furthermore, in the non-ginseng period of time, his performance dropped back to its usual rate, confirming that ginseng was the cause of his increased energy. (This fall in performance is due to the high dosage taken during the intense trial period.) Eric explained that in each three-week test period, it usually took about four or five days to see the improvement in his performance, but then it was immediately clear that he had begun to experience a jump in his output which lasted the duration of the trial period. Eric said that the ginseng kept his heart rate lower during both trials and increased the wattage of his output.

Eric has continued taking ginseng since late 1995, and he attributes a significant improvement in his performance to it. He is convinced that taking ginseng has allowed his body to exert more energy and to recover more quickly after training sessions. As Eric points out, serious athletes who work out extensively develop a high level of sensitivity to what happens inside their bodies; they can literally feel their bodies' metabolism and can tell if their bodies are working at their maximum. In this sense, Eric is convinced that his body is in much better shape because of the ginseng. He also points out that since adding ginseng to his diet, he has not been sick once, which is very unusual for most athletes, who often get sick immediately before or after competition from the stress of the competition and from the extreme physical demands they put on their bodies.

Eric told me that he intends to continue taking ginseng because he is so confident of the results it provides. Along with the ginseng, he also takes an L-argenine supplement before going to bed to help his metabolism become more efficient, and a thermogenics supplement that helps his body burn more calories to reduce the level of fat in his body. All these supplements, including ginseng, are natural products and are admissible nutritional supplements in sporting competitions. Eric is currently entering about twelve triathlon competitions a year, and each triathlon typically includes a 1.5-kilometer swim, a 40-kilometer bike race, and a 10-kilometer marathon. Some triathlons are even more strenuous, such as the famous Iron Man triathlon in Hawaii, which includes a 2.4-mile swim, a 112-mile bike race, and a full 26.2-mile marathon run.

The Chemistry of Excellent Performance

What accounts for ginseng's ability to improve one's physical performance in terms of normal workload, or in athletics? In simple terms, the answer again lies in the fact that ginseng moderates the body's stress response. Because the body reacts more quickly and efficiently to cope with any stressor, including increased physical demand, it experiences less stress, and this translates into an improvement in your body's ability to meet physical challenges.

More specifically, the link between the stress response and an increase in your body's ability to perform physically may be traced directly to ginseng's influence on the hormonal system, particularly in initially stimulating the adrenal glands. There are several reasons why ginseng aids your body in this way. First, when you engage in any physical performance, your body consumes energy from the fuel stored in muscle tissues and from the sugars in the bloodstream. It is precisely the adrenal glands and the hormones which these glands produce that control the energy consumption process during periods of heavy demand. This physiological connection suggests that ginseng gives your body the initial energy boost it needs when called on to perform physically.

Second, the adrenal hormones are also involved in many other metabolic processes necessary for lasting physical strength and aerobic endurance, such as increasing your heart rate, dilating the blood vessels in the muscle tissues, controlling your blood pressure, and regulating the salt and water balance in your body. Because ginseng helps to moderate the adrenal gland's hormonal production, you gain endurance and stamina. With better control of your heart rate, blood flow, and salt/water balance in your blood, your body is able to withstand for longer periods of time the demands placed upon it.

Ginseng's role in enhancing your endurance is especially critical during strenuous, heart-thumping, oxygen-demanding physical work or sports. This is because when your body is physically taxed to an extreme, it undergoes a critical metabolic change from an *aerobic* metabolism to an *anaerobic* metabolism. According to Eric Harr, the body's aerobic metabolism is thirty-nine times more efficient than its anaerobic metabolism. Furthermore, when your muscles begin working anaerobically, they produce more lactic acid, a chemical that creates the pain and fatigue in muscle tissue. The longer you can work out in an aerobic state, the better it is for your body; your muscles are more efficient in using energy, and they produce less of the debilitating lactic acid. This means that the longer you are able to delay the transition from aerobic to anaerobic by reducing your heart rate, breathing rate, and oxygen usage, the more endurance you will have, and the better your performance will be. This is precisely what ginseng accomplishes for you!

Researchers also believe that ginseng directly influences the body's production and use of energy at the cellular level, although this too may occur because of its influence on the hormonal production in the adrenal glands. You have probably heard the terms *anabolic* and *catabolic*. Anabolic refers to how cells produce energy, and catabolic refers to the process of using up this energy. Ginseng appears to play a role in improving both sides of the equation:

Anabolic

Research suggests that ginseng helps the body make more sparing use of carbohydrates when you work out. It also helps the body rebuild its energy reserves of glycogen and high-energy phosphorous compounds in the liver. Both of these actions contribute to greater endurance. Some of the biochemical evidence for this suggests that ginseng influences the production of ATPase, the enzyme that helps transform food molecules to ATP, which is the fuel used by the body's cells. Ginseng has also been shown to increase the synthesis of RNA in the nucleus and cytoplasm of rat liver cells. In humans, these same liver cells are responsible for the production of energy from amino acids broken down from food. This means that ginseng likely improves the way your body produces and uses its reserves of energy in the liver.

Catabolic

Ginseng also seems to play a role in preserving the health of muscle tissue during periods of heavy usage. This occurs because ginseng affects the liver cells that manage the absorption of lactic acid produced by activated muscles. When too much lactic acid builds up in the muscles, they become fatigued and sore. With ginseng, the liver cells absorb greater amounts of lactic acid (which is transformed back to glucose), thus reducing muscle aches and pains.

It's All Natural

One of the most critical points to understand about ginseng and its influence on your body's metabolism is that it does so in natural ways, unlike synthetic drugs that are commonly used to increase energy and endurance. The most well-known of these drugs are anabolic steroids, which, as you probably have heard, pump up the steroidal hormones in the body to such dangerous levels that severe physiological damage often results. Anabolic steroids are banned from every major competitive sport, including the Olympics. Although anabolic steroids build up the body's muscle tissue and energy supplies, they throw the body's hormonal system out of whack. Male athletes who use anabolic steroids typically exhibit abnormal muscle growth far beyond their natural proportions, as well as a dangerous increase in their heart rate and blood pressure. Female athletes who use anabolic steroids may undergo severe side effects related to an increase in testosterone, which causes a deepening of the voice, hair growth, and changes in body tone that make the female physique look more masculine. In recent years, several athletes who had been using anabolic steroids to improve their conditioning have died as a result of the destructive nature of the steroids on their bodies' hormonal system.

In contrast, ginseng is not associated with any negative side effects, because it appears to interact with the body's hypothalamus/pituitary/adrenal axis very naturally at a very low level. To prove this, several experiments have been conducted on athletes who were given ginseng for fourteen days; they were given urine tests to ascertain if there were traces of any "doping" substances in their bodies. Doping substances are residues of illegal stimulants and muscle builders that have been banned by the International Olympic Committee. In every experiment, ginseng left no doping traces at all, indicating that its active ingredients are absorbed so entirely in the body and at such a deep molecular level that it leaves no footprint at all. In contrast, stimulants such as amphetamines, anabolic steroids, and even nicotine and caffeine can be traced in the body for many months after their usage.

Improving Mental Performance Too

Even if sports or physical endurance are not major components in your life, you can benefit from ginseng because it also appears to have an equally important effect in enhancing your mental performance. Over the course of many research experiments, ginseng has been shown to speed up people's reflexes and to enhance their learning faculties. Here is a short list of several of the most noted experiments in this area:

- In several Soviet studies of telegraph operators who were given assignments to test their ability to work quickly, those who had been given ginseng improved the accuracy of their work.

- In a double-blind study involving male volunteers between the ages of twenty and twenty-four, the group that had taken ginseng extract for twelve weeks had greater levels of attention, arithmetic mental processing, coordination, and faster auditory reaction times than the placebo group.

- In a German study of sixty people, ages twenty to seventy, half of the subjects were given a ginseng extract. Both groups were tested for visual acuity by using a flickering light test in which the subjects were asked to determine at what point they could no longer distinguish a quickly flickering light (i.e., as the light flickers faster and faster, it eventually looks like a continuous light). The group given ginseng had a higher threshold of visual acuity after twelve weeks, meaning they could see individual light flickers for longer than the control group. In the same experiment, the subjects were also given visual and auditory response time tests in which they had to react to visual and sound stimuli; again, those given ginseng had a more significant improvement in their reaction times over twelve weeks. These same groups were also given two-handed coordination tests, and once again, the group given ginseng had a higher degree of improvement in their coordination over the twelve weeks of ginseng administration.

▣ There have also been hundreds of animal studies (using mice and rats) that have shown substantial increases in learning ability. In one of the most well-known animal studies, university researchers in Japan placed rats in a simple "Y" maze; after being released, the rats had to choose between two different paths—one leading to a reward, the other to nothing. The rat's rate of learning was then measured by the number of trials it took for the animal to learn which alley contained the food reward. In some of these experiments, the rats were given either ginseng or caffeine. To the surprise of the researchers, the rats that were given ginseng had considerably shorter learning times than the rats that were given caffeine. The rats that were given caffeine also tired more quickly. In another study, rats were trained to climb a pole or jump over a barrier whenever a tone was sounded (so as to avoid a mildly annoying shock); those treated with ginseng learned to respond more rapidly to the tone than did a control group.

◉ At this time, the biology behind the mental and learning improvements attributed to ginseng are not as well understood as the physical enhancements, largely because research on how the brain functions is still at a rather primitive stage. Some research suggests that ginseng excites the nervous system—particularly Asian ginseng because of its higher level of Rg1 ginsenosides. Other research has speculated that the chemical *choline*, which performs many important functions in the body and is found in ginseng, may also contribute to the process. Choline lowers the blood pressure and seems to improve memory in patients suffering from senility.

◉ In addition, several other experiments have provided another indirect clue to how ginseng may work in the brain. In these experiments, the subjects suffered from a lack of blood flow to the brain. In one experiment, forty-five subjects were given either a pharmaceutical drug, ginseng, or a placebo. The group that received the pharmaceutical drug had a 58% improvement in blood flow, which was not surprising, but the ginseng group improved their blood flow by 34%, compared to less than 1% for the placebo group. In another experiment, 170 patients between the ages of forty-one and seventy received two capsules of ginseng extract a day. Of these patients, 36% had very favorable improvements in blood flow in the carotid artery and in the brain, while 54% had small improvements in the elasticity of their arteries and blood flow. These results suggest that ginseng heightens the blood flow in the brain, helping to nourish brain cells with fresh supplies of energy.

▣ Scientists also know that the hormones released in many endocrine system glands play a role in brain function and may influence the central nervous system, but the precise mechanisms by which this happens are not fully understood. One possible link is through the control of many blood chemicals that are needed by the nervous system, such as potassium and sodium. Since ginseng helps the adrenals, whose hormones regulate the chemical content of the blood, ginseng may thus have an indirect beneficial effect on the brain.

Getting the Edge

The implications of years of research overwhelmingly indicate a solid correlation between ginseng and enhanced physical and mental performance. At this point, there can be no doubt that the benefits of a regular supplement of ginseng can be enormous, affecting all the activities in which you participate day in and day out. In terms of physical performance, whether you are doing hard physical labor, taking part in a rigorous competitive sport, or simply enjoying an afternoon game of golf, you will find that your ability to exert yourself harder and for longer periods of time increases, while the feelings of strain and pain in your body decrease. In terms of mental performance, you will notice a significant improvement in your ability to focus and concentrate on intellectual tasks, and an uplift in your mood and attitude, both of which can greatly influence your success in solving problems and challenges.

On the basis of the vast amount of research that has been done, it is important to note that ginseng appears to help people of all types. As shown by experiments cited in this chapter, tests of ginseng have been performed in many different countries with test subjects varying in age and physical condition. Although in a few of the tests the results were not uniform for all age groups (with the best results achieved by the most fit or the least fit test subjects in the fifty-plus age range), in general the benefits of ginseng in most tests apply across the board to all population groups. Nevertheless, it is clear that more research would be useful to determine if certain ages or populations are more sensitive to substantial improvements, mentally or physically.

In my own practice, I have recommended ginseng to hundreds of my patients, who have all returned to me feeling a renewed sense of vim and vigor in their lives, often within one month. In fact, most people to whom I recommend ginseng have reported the same results in terms of greater endurance and stamina, particularly while engaged in physical activities. One couple of thirty-year-olds that I've worked with, Dan and Jane Gilmond, both use ginseng to boost their energy all day long. When asked how much he liked using ginseng, Dan told me, "My wife swears by it, and I now feel it helps me too. I am not the type of person who normally takes any medications, not even an aspirin for a headache. But my wife suggested that I start using it because I am in the construction industry, which requires me to have a lot of energy all day long. I find that ginseng makes me feel peppy all day long. In particular, it also helps me get rid of what I call 'the lazy effect' in the morning. By this I mean that I used to be slow at getting moving in the morning; now I take ginseng first thing, and I can get moving."

A forty-five-year-old male patient, Rick Benzel, came to me because he was just starting to work out regularly after almost two decades of only occasional exercise and a poor diet, which had left him ten pounds overweight. He began a daily regimen of Siberian ginseng supplements to boost his energy and noticed results within one month. Rick told me that before taking ginseng, playing three sets of tennis or bicycling for sixty minutes wore him down almost to the point of complete exhaustion. Once, however, he began taking two capsules of ginseng each day, his lung capacity began increasing and his endurance improved to the point where an hour of either activity did not leave him dazed or breathless. Naturally, the sheer fact of getting more exercise also contributed to his improvement, but, as Rick himself says, the ginseng was instrumental in increasing his strength and stamina.

Another patient, Brian Crocker, is a thirty-two-year-old amateur golfer who has been practicing for ten years with the goal of becoming a professional golfer. At my recommendation, Brian began taking ginseng more than four years ago, and now attributes a significant improvement in his golf game to ginseng. In fact, he recently became a finalist in the California State Amateur Golf Championship. Brian told me, "I take Siberian ginseng once a day; sometimes I even take two in the morning. I find that ginseng especially gives me energy around midday, when I normally start to feel tired and listless. In terms of my golf game, I've noticed that ginseng helps me feel great from the beginning of a round to the end; it literally keeps my energy flowing the entire time. In fact, when I forget to take ginseng for a day or two, I actually notice a drop in my energy level. I also feel that ginseng helps my mental performance; I concentrate better and stay focused on my game. Golf is a very mental and emotional game. If your body isn't feeling good, you can't play well. I really think ginseng helps me feel better. Since I've been using ginseng, I've been playing better golf than I've ever played before."

If you are interested in getting the edge on your physical and mental performance, it is worth your serious consideration to try ginseng for a month and then examine your results. Depending on certain factors such as your diet, your current physical condition, and your attitude, you will likely see some degree of improvement, whether you are playing a sport or performing mentally for your work. In either case, you can be sure that the addition of ginseng to your diet will be responsible for the change.

Ginseng and Your Sex Life

Can one desire too much of a good thing?

William Shakespeare
(1564–1616), English
dramatist and poet

The discussion of performance in the last chapter naturally leads us to a related topic: sex. Indeed, romance is perhaps the one area of life in which most of us take our capacity seriously, believing that when we get into bed with our partner, we need to function at our best.

Most people will probably admit that they do not make love as well or as often as they would like. For many couples, the stresses and pressures of life drain their sex drive and cause them to be worn down and fatigued at day's end. Physical intimacy is usually the farthest thing from their mind when they go to bed at night. Even in the morning when they wake up, they usually feel pressured to focus immediately on their kids or on getting ready to go to work. Many couples can go for weeks without having sex, and this abstinence compounds their problem even more. A lack of sex often engenders a vicious circle in which the partners begin to feel emotionally detached or resentful, and this leads to feelings of isolation, greater detachment, and so on and so on.

Even when they make love, many couples are disappointed by the level of enjoyment they derive from it. First, their stress and fatigue often make their lovemaking a short, single event rather than a prolonged experience that includes ample time for mutual foreplay and intimate cuddling. The stress of performance may drain the partners emotionally, so they cannot focus on each other in stimulating, loving ways, or the partners may be so physically exhausted or even out of shape that coupling for a long period of time is simply beyond their capacity. In fact, it is estimated that the average lovemaking session for a typical couple is only between five and ten minutes.

In addition, the partners may also suffer from various physical or emotional ailments that prevent their intimate moments from being as dynamic and pleasurable as they might be. For example, some men have problems developing or maintaining a satisfactory erection that pleases their partner, or may produce only a small amount of semen, so that their orgasm is short-lived or even painful. Women, too, can suffer from a lack of lubrication, which makes lovemaking arduous and unpleasurable. Certain physical ailments and diseases significantly interfere with sex as well. These include diabetes and prostatitis in men, and vaginitis, urinary tract infections, and PMS in women.

If any of these issues sound familiar to you, this chapter will show you how ginseng can make a major difference in your sexual life. Whether it is stress, fatigue, lack of sex drive, or certain types of physical ailments that are taking a toll on your relationship, you will see how adding ginseng to your diet—and your partner's diet—can give both of you a renewed sense of energy so that you can capture the heightened pleasure you would like to have.

Aphrodisiacs—Myth Versus Fact

You may be thinking at this point that I am going to reiterate the ancient idea that ginseng helps your sex life because it is an "aphrodisiac," i.e., a substance that stimulates or prolongs sexual desire. As pointed out earlier in the book, this has long been one of the most common perceptions about ginseng, dating as far back as several thousand years ago, when it was believed that the penis-like shape of the root implied that it had special properties to endow men with superior sexual energy and vitality. One might even say that the vast folklore behind ginseng as an aphrodisiac is responsible for spreading the word about the herb throughout the world. It is an undeniable fact that nearly every culture that has grown ginseng—from India and Korea to England and France, and even among the Native American tribes—has cherished it for its reputed sexual empowerment.

However, in our culture, accepting the concept of aphrodisiacs is difficult for most people. The fact that other cultures have so fiercely touted them is of no consequence to us, since we tend to think of other cultures as primitive and unsophisticated in their knowledge of science and medicine. The notion that ginseng's shape has anything to do with the potency of a male's penis makes us chuckle. In our world, the image of an aphrodisiac typically brings to mind such things as a medieval witches' brew made from bizarre items like dog's hair, goat's blood, and a lizard's tail, or perhaps a plate of oysters and a glass of wine.

There can be no doubt that a great deal of hype or myth lies behind many aphrodisiacs. But given the primacy of love and sex to our species, it is actually quite natural that people throughout the ages have wanted to test their local herbs and foodstuffs to learn if any of them might spur sexual vitality and attraction. Concocting "creative" mixtures of exotic and erotic items is also quite normal, if not clever; after all, isn't that what the greatest chefs from time immemorial have done to perfect what we now consider *haute cuisine*?

It's not hard to imagine how an aphrodisiac came to be discovered or invented; all that was needed was one man or woman to ingest some herb or concoction, followed by a few hours of an uncontrollable sexual appetite and passionate lovemaking, for the word to spread. Of course, the problem is that in the past there was little scientific evidence to prove or disprove a linkage between the herb or concoction and the increased sexual capacity. People simply took it on faith when a person in their village howled about having great sex the night before after ingesting something his wife had made.

Ironically, the effectiveness of some purported aphrodisiacs in history may actually lie in what modern science calls the "placebo effect"; that is, if an individual takes something he or she *thinks* is an aphrodisiac, it actually works. The mind convinces the body that the substance causes great lovemaking, and thus it does. The placebo effect is very well known and accepted in modern medicine and in some instances a placebo pill has been known to actually cure people of diseases or put them into remission, even though they have received no medicine. An amazing example of the placebo effect can be found on a box of Rogaine, the liquid now being sold over the counter to stimulate hair growth in bald men. According to the manufacturer, Upjohn, while Rogaine helped 26% of the experimental male subjects regrow hair, 11% of those who used a placebo liquid also sprouted hair. How's that for demonstrating the power of wishful thinking!

Modern scientists first discovered the powerful link between the body and the mind when they were studying the "fight or flight" syndrome. When you are in a situation that causes you to feel fear, your body gears up for the stress response: your endocrine system releases adrenaline into the bloodstream, your blood pressure and rate of breathing increases, and your muscles become tense. However, scientists noticed that an individual does not have to be actually threatened to elicit these physical responses of fear. All it takes is for the brain to think you are in danger, and the body will react. The mind convinces the body that danger is near, and the body initiates the fight-or-flight response.

The same mind/body effect occurs with many alleged aphrodisiacs. When your brain thinks that a substance or ritual will sexually enhance the body, it will trigger the flow of the hormones and chemicals that prepare you for sex and enhance your performance. This placebo effect probably explains the effect of many a witch's brew throughout history of giving men larger, harder erections or for turning their lovers into insatiable nymphomaniacs. Modern people are clearly not immune to the mind/body effect, so if you take ginseng or any other reputed aphrodisiac thinking that it can contribute to your sexual capabilities, it very likely will.

The Chemistry of Aphrodisiacs

This is not to suggest that ginseng or other aphrodisiacs work solely because of the placebo effect. In fact, researchers are increasingly recognizing that many substances, including ginseng, actually contribute in real physiological or chemical ways to improving a person's sexual health and capabilities. To see how this is so, it is necessary to first clarify two issues about human sex.

First, the sexual process is much more complicated than most of us realize. Sex can be divided into four phases: desire, arousal, orgasm, and male ejaculation. All four of these phases must take place in synchronicity within each person and between the two partners for a successful sexual encounter to occur. A problem in any one area can prevent intercourse from occurring or cause it to occur only with pain and displeasure. For example, some people may suffer from a lack of desire caused by a chemical imbalance in their brain cells, by a physical disease, or by an emotional ailment such as depression. Others cannot get aroused, such as men who have erection problems or women who have vaginal infections. Still others can-

not achieve orgasm or ejaculation for various psychological and physiological reasons.

Second, all four phases involve the coordination of
many mind/body systems. What most of us noncha-
lantly refer to as "sexual chemistry" is actually quite
complex. When you meet someone new and secretly
size him or her up as a sexual partner, or when you
look into your spouse's eyes with those bedroom
thoughts, there is actually an amazing array of events
happening inside the body. The following bodily systems must function properly for pleasurable, rewarding
intimacy to occur:

▣ The body's autonomic nervous system (the com-
mand center that regulates unconscious activity) is
critical in preparing you for sex. Just as during the
fight-or-flight response, when you become aroused
there is a fine interplay between the sympathetic
and parasympathetic branches of the autonomic
nervous system. In the beginning, arousal causes the
parasympathetic system to take over; the brain produces acetylcholine, the blood vessels dilate, and
blood pressure drops. This provides an erection for
the man and clitoral excitation for the woman. As
orgasm approaches, the body switches to the sympathetic nervous system, which floods the body with
adrenaline and other hormones. The blood vessels
constrict, the heart rate increases, blood pressure
rises, and orgasm and ejaculation occur.

▣ The endocrine system (based in the pituitary/hypo-thalamus/adrenal axis) produces three hormones that prepare the body for intercourse. Without the balanced production of these hormones, any one of the four sexual phases may suffer. Testosterone, produced in both men and women but in greater amounts in men, is the hormone that fuels the libido, stimulating the sex drive needed to initiate desire. Estrogen, also produced in both men and women but in greater amounts in women, affects the emotions and mood during arousal. In women, estrogen also produces the lubrication in the vaginal walls needed for comfortable penetration. The third hormone, progesterone, is also secreted by both genders, and in women it stimulates the lining of the uterus in preparation for impregnation.

▣ The brain's neurotransmitters play a critical role in the phases of the sexual process. The chemical *dopamine* is the "alertness" neurotransmitter and is needed for the libido; dopamine is what gets you aroused and excited. The neurotransmitter *serotonin*, produced in the brain from tryptophan, is necessary to trigger orgasm. Similarly, the neuropeptides produced in the brain and the body are also required for pleasure and arousal. One neuropeptide, abbreviated VIP (vasoactive intestinal peptide), is believed to work on the dilation of the blood vessels that cause the male erection. Another neuropeptide, *oxytocin*, has been linked to the contractions during orgasm in both men and women. (In fact, you may know that synthesized oxytocin is sometimes given to women during childbirth because it stimulates uterine contractions.)

▣ Finally, the sex act itself also involves the body's muscular system, particularly in the abdominal and pelvic areas, but in other muscle groups as well, depending on the position used during lovemaking.

Given the complexity of the sexual response and the number of bodily systems involved, it has become increasingly clear to modern science that sexual health is a delicate affair. To have a "healthy" sexual response, i.e., one that allows you to have the proper mood and sensitive feelings, as well as arousal and orgasm, your body must be in tune, and all its sexual systems must be properly nourished and energized. The brain, the nervous and endocrine systems, and the muscles must have received the care and nourishment needed to generate the hormones, neurotransmitters, and neuropeptides required for a healthy sexual response. These bodily systems are directly fueled by the foods you eat; the muscles, hormones, neurotransmitters, and neuropeptides are built out of the vitamins, minerals, and amino acids you ingest in foods. Many factors, such as a poor diet, disease, or a chemical imbalance in the endocrine system or brain can completely disable the sexual response. Fatigue, diseases such as diabetes, and emotional problems such as depression can literally halt your interest in sex or your ability to perform it.

This is precisely how aphrodisiacs fit in. Aphrodisiacs are actually nothing more than substances that have a significant or immediate effect in nourishing or restoring the body's endocrine and chemical sexual systems. Whereas ancient cultures believed that aphrodisiacs were magic, modern science can now attribute their effectiveness to a greater understanding of sexual chemistry. Some substances work to stimulate our desire (libido) by feeding the brain's neurotransmitters and neuropeptides or help with arousal, orgasm, or ejaculation by feeding the hormonal system. Other substances simply prevent us from becoming sick or succumbing to a disease or emotional problem that blocks healthy sexuality.

In her book *Love Potions: A Guide to Aphrodisiacs and Sexual Pleasures*, Dr. Cynthia Watson, M.D., writes:

Myth and legends notwithstanding, some foods definitely have a physiological role in human desire. The sex drive requires a balance between the endocrine and neurologic systems, and the foods that are the most sexually stimulating contain nutrients that support these systems. The endocrine system needs nourishment to supply the building blocks for hormones; the neurologic system needs the same for production of neuro-transmitters and neuropeptides. Ideally, you should get these nutrients—vitamins, minerals, amino acids, essential fatty acids, mucopolysac-charides, and glandulars—from a normal diet. At the very least, a sexually dynamic body needs a diet rich in fresh and varied fruits and vegetables and lean animal protein or legumes.

Watson goes on to list many foods and herbs that are particularly rich in vitamins, minerals, amino acids, and fatty acids that empower and enrich our body's sexual systems. Some of these substances work on the endocrine system, and some on the neurotransmitters and neuropeptides. In many cases, these foods and herbs are exactly those that one or more ancient cultures perceived as aphrodisiacs, even though they did not have the science to prove it. For example, oysters have long been considered an aphrodisiac in many cultures. We now know that oysters are extremely high in zinc and complex sugars and proteins, all of which are important to the health of the male prostate gland, which secretes the seminal fluid that mixes with se-men to form a male's ejaculate. In other words, eating oysters literally does enhance ejaculation. Similarly, asparagus was often thought of as an aphrodisiac, partially because of its phallic nature and partially from the lore that surrounded it as a sexual performance enhancer. We now know that it contains large amounts of vitamin E, which is required for the production of the adrenal hormones that are critical to the sexual response. Another common ancient aphrodisiac was honey; again, we now know that honey contains high amounts of B-complex vitamins and minerals, which promote sexual health in both men and women. Even chocolate turns out to have a real chemical rationale behind its name, the "lover's food." Chocolate contains the amino acid *phenylalanine*, which increases the level of the pleasure-inducing neuropeptide *phenylethylamine* in the brain. This is why eating chocolate makes lovers feel good about each other; they are high from the neuropeptides in their brains.

Research into several exotic "high-powered" aphrodisiacs — those that make men feel they can ejaculate several times or that give women the sense they can have multiple orgasms — has also proven that many of them truly do work because they reinforce the body's endocrine or nervous system. For example, the African herb *yohimbine*, which is derived from the bark of the yohimbé tree, dilates small arteries because it blocks the release of a neurotransmitter that controls artery constriction. This then causes an increase of blood flow to the penis and clitoris, which provides more sensitivity and, in men, harder erections. Unfortunately, it is also known that yohimbine may have serious side effects, including nausea, heart palpitations, excessive perspiration, tension, and irritability. Another exotic aphrodisiac, *damiana*, which grows in Mexico and Texas, contains several alkaloids that directly stimulate the nerves and sex organs, increase circulation, and have a muscle-relaxing effect. Some research also shows that damiana increases sperm count in men.

Ginseng, Aphrodisiacs, and Sex

How then does ginseng fit into this view of aphrodisiacs and the body's complex sexual systems? Is ginseng a sexual placebo, or does it have real effects on the body?

The answer is found in the chemical makeup of ginseng. Because of the ginsenosides (eleutherosides in Siberian ginseng), vitamins, and trace minerals in ginseng, we now know that it has a wide range of generalized tonic effects on the body. As an adaptogen, ginseng balances the entire body, normalizing the functioning of many bodily systems. If your body is suffering from high blood pressure, it lowers it; if you have low blood sugar, ginseng helps to raise it. In this way, ginseng makes your entire body healthier and provides you with a significantly greater capacity for activity of any kind, including sex. After all, sex is extremely demanding on the mind and body, and just as ginseng improves your performance in sports or physical labor, it also allows your body to answer the call of sex with greater stamina and endurance.

Because ginseng (especially Chinese and Korean ginseng) is a stimulant, some people benefit sexually because they feel a much higher level of alertness and a resistance to fatigue after taking ginseng. Rather than feeling stressed out and exhausted at night, they are more likely to be interested in lovemaking. Ginseng gives them the added alertness and motivation to engage in sex when they otherwise would have wanted to "veg out" on the couch.

Ginseng can also be considered a true aphrodisiac because its chemical makeup has measurable positive effects on the body's endocrine system. Through its actions in boosting the adrenal glands, ginseng directly reinforces the production of your body's sexual hormones elaborated in that gland: testosterone, estrogen, and progesterone. Because your adrenals are less taxed, your body is also able to maintain a better balance in the production of hormones and to make them continually, even if you engage in sex several times a day. In this sense, the correlation between ginseng and sexual prowess is quite direct.

Although no formal human studies have focused on ginseng and sex, a broad range of animal experiments have confirmed these beneficial effects on sexual function. In several different tests conducted by many different researchers, ginseng speeded up the sexual maturity of mice and rabbits, increased semen production in bulls, reduced the number of sterile females among mink, and increased the blood levels of prolactin, a hormone that stimulates the production of progesterone in the ovaries. In other experiments, the weight of the prostate gland and seminal vesicles increased among male mice when they were given ginseng, and female mice that were given ginseng had an increase in the length of periods of sexual activity.

Taken together, the nonspecific effects of ginseng on the body as a whole and the specific effects on the endocrine system go far to justify the myth that ginseng is truly an aphrodisiac. By making your body healthier in general, ginseng can enhance your entire sexual functioning. It makes you feel better, increases your desire, heightens your ability to get aroused, and improves your performance by giving you and your partner stamina and endurance. Meanwhile, by directly affecting your endocrine system, ginseng also helps to regulate one of the most critical sexual systems in the body, giving you a healthier libido (via regulation of testosterone) and better moods (via regulation of estrogen).

Sex is obviously a very private and subjective experience, but I have received dozens of anecdotal reports from my patients and others confirming amazing results from the addition of ginseng to their diets. Many men, ranging in age from their twenties to forties, told me that they experienced a significant increase in their desire, and a few of the men reported a noticeable increase in the amount of semen and seminal fluid they ejaculated. Many women told me that after taking ginseng for just a few days, their desire for sex increased, and their ability to achieve a full orgasm flowered. In several cases, healthy married women who had lost their desire for sex after having children reported to me that ginseng renewed their interest in sex for the first time since childbirth. One of my favorite cases involved a man of sixty-plus years who began taking ginseng just to see what would happen; he returned to me after just a few days and thanked me profusely on behalf of his wife, who said ginseng had rejuvenated their relationship.

An Antidote to Alcohol

Another curious side effect of ginseng that indirectly relates to sex is the beneficial effect it seems to have on the body's intake of alcohol. Research has shown that ginseng moderates the effects of alcohol and sedative drugs in the body. The way ginseng does this is not precisely known, but it appears to be related to the effect ginseng has on glycogen levels in the liver, which is the organ that rids the body of alcohol. The sequence of events is as follows: alcohol is absorbed from the intestine into the bloodstream, where it is carried to the liver, which metabolizes it by breaking it down. However, when you consume more than about an ounce of alcohol per hour, the liver cannot keep up, so the alcohol remains in your bloodstream, where it invades your fat cells and other organs. After about three drinks, your entire body begins to suffer; because your blood has a high alcohol content, the nerve cells in your brain are dulled and cannot properly transmit or receive neurotransmitter chemicals to your other organs and your muscles. As a result, you become uncoordinated and agitated, and your performance is severely diminished—including your ability to have sex!

Taking ginseng, however, improves the liver's ability to handle the alcohol. In one experiment, subjects who had taken ginseng had 35% lower blood alcohol levels than the control group, which had not taken ginseng prior to drinking. This moderating effect can be an advantage in our culture, where alcohol and romance often go hand in hand. In the Western view, alcohol is perceived as an aphrodisiac because it lowers inhibitions and generally makes people more willing to engage in sexual play. Too much alcohol, however, nullifies the loss of inhibition. This is because alcohol sedates the central nervous system and interferes with erection and orgasm. As Shakespeare wrote, alcohol "provokes the desire but takes away the performance."

In this sense, ginseng may help some people keep the flames burning after drinking. In general though, the less alcohol you have before engaging in sex, the better your performance and endurance will be. In fact, excessive alcohol usage can have serious side effects on your sexuality. In men, chronic alcohol abuse lowers the libido and suppresses the production of testosterone in the testes. In women, chronic use of alcohol can have a toxic effect on the ovaries and can even cause infertility by blocking the hypothalamus/pituitary release of hormones. Research shows that women alcoholics usually reach menopause earlier than women who drink only moderately or not at all.

Fertility, Pregnancy, and Ginseng

There may also be some relationship between ginseng and fertility, although more research is needed in this area. This potential connection is due to the fact that the regulation of progesterone in women can contribute to improved fertility. Progesterone levels are highest in women during the second half of their menstrual cycle because the hormone stimulates the uterine lining in preparation for pregnancy. Since ginseng supports the adrenals, it may be that the regulation of progesterone is one of its beneficial effects.

As for pregnancy, the consumption of ginseng during pregnancy has long been the tradition in China, where it is believed that ginseng supplies extra energy for the fetus. In a study of eighty-eight women who took ginseng during their pregnancies, there was a lower incidence of preeclampsia (a form of toxemia in pregnancy) among those women who took ginseng than among those in the control group.

Nevertheless, at this point in the research on ginseng, *it is not recommended that you take ginseng if you are pregnant or nursing a baby without first consulting your physician.* Korean or Chinese red ginseng, a strong stimulant, is especially to be avoided.

Jump-Start Your Sex Life with Ginseng

So if you and your mate suffer from low sex drive, or your sexual engagements are disappointing and lackluster, ginseng can truly help. Of course, it is best if both partners begin taking ginseng simultaneously, but even if only one of you takes it, you will likely find within a matter of days that your romantic interactions become more vigorous, if not more frequent. Given that poor sex is often a contributory factor behind the failure of many relationships, ginseng is certainly worth a try. You might also read Dr. Cynthia Watson's book, *Love Potions*, for ideas on how to set up a wonderfully sensual evening, complete with aromatic scents, erotic foods, and fragrant massage oils that will incite and delight your passions.

Naturally, ginseng cannot solve deep emotional problems that may occur between mates. If your sexual problems reflect more serious relationship issues, no aphrodisiac in this world will help you more than temporarily. Also, ginseng cannot inflame passions between strangers, so don't go running off thinking that if you give a ginseng pill to a potential partner, sex will happen that night. If it does, congratulate yourself, but don't ascribe the lust to the ginseng; it is really the chemistry between the two of you that inspired it. If sex doesn't happen—the more likely result—don't blame the ginseng. This is where the belief in magical aphrodisiacs that create instant sex becomes pure fantasy. No herbal product can instill the sexual urge in someone who does not already have it.

In addition to adding ginseng to your diet, I recommend that you also consult the following chart, which lists some of most important nutritional substances that you need to emphasize in your diet to have a healthier sex life. By eating more of the foods that contain these vitamins and minerals, you will discover that your sexual health will be greatly enhanced.

Element Vitamins	Need/Use	Where Found	Comments
B-1 Thiamin	Essential for healthy heart, muscles, adrenal glands, fertility	Soybeans, beans, peas, peanuts, whole-grain breads, asparagus, raw nuts, yogurt	Low levels of B-1 may be associated with depression and anorexia
B-2 Riboflavin	Required for red blood cell production; keeps hair and skin healthy; helps body obtain energy from carbohydrates and proteins	Asparagus, bananas, figs, whole grains, green vegetables, lean meats, eggs	
B-3 Niacin	Combats anxiety, depression, insomnia, and fatigue; dilates blood vessels; essential for synthesis of sex hormones	Fish, lean meats, peas, beans, avocados, figs, dates, whole-grain cereals, asparagus	Niacin supplements can irritate stomach; start with doses of 100 milligrams, not to exceed 2 grams per day

Element Vitamins	Need/Use	Where Found	Comments
B-5 Pantothenic acid	Known as stress vitamin; healthy functioning of adrenal gland and the production of steroid hormones	Nuts, grains, eggs, beef, potatoes, broccoli, cabbage, bee pollen	Helps combat aging and for menopausal women
B-12	Production of red blood cells; required for digestion, protein synthesis, and metabolism	Fish, shellfish, seaweed, milk, cheese, eggs	Strict vegetarians may need to take a supplement
Choline	Required by brain to produce neurotransmitter acetylcholine which is essential to nervous system	Egg yolks, seeds, grains, nuts, soybeans, meats, poultry, green vegetables	Recent research has linked lack of choline and Alzheimer's disease
Lecithin	Prevents cell membranes from hardening; makes up protective sheath surrounding the brain	Brewer's yeast, whole grains, legumes, and fish	Large amounts secreted in semen; needs to be replaced after ejaculation

Element *Vitamins*	Need/Use	Where Found	Comments
Folic acid	Necessary for energy production and formation of red blood cells	Salmon, tuna, green leafy vegetables, root vegetables, whole grains, cheese, oranges	Research has found this to be important in preventing birth defects; also believed to be an antiaging vitamin
Vitamin A (retinol)	Needed for new cell growth, healthy tissue, and vision in dim light; also for healthy production of sperm, and for healthy thyroid gland	Body converts carotene found in carrots, yams, and pumpkins to Vitamin A. Retinol found in liver, eggs, milk	Vitamin A used in tandem with Vitamin E to raise sperm count
Vitamin C (ascorbic acid)	Promotes tissue growth, bone healing, and is important for adrenal and pituitary glands; protects against free radical damage from pollutants	Citrus fruits, kiwi, tomatoes, bell peppers, kale, green vegetables	Also important for formation of collagen, which helps keep skin supple and elastic

Element *Vitamins*	Need/Use	Where Found	Comments
Vitamin E	Required for production of hormones and prostaglandins, to repair cells, and as an antioxidant	Vegetable oils, nuts, seeds, beans, eggs, whole grains, fruits, asparagus, peas	Often referred to as the "sex" vitamin
Minerals			
Zinc	Important for healthy male sexuality, needed for production of testosterone	Oysters, legumes, pumpkin seeds, garlic, spinach	Zinc supplements have been shown to help with prostatitis; when taking zinc, be sure to get enough copper from green vegetables
Calcium	Essential for strong bones, teeth, and muscles	Salmon, sardines, seaweed, green leafy vegetables, almonds	Women need calcium to prevent osteoporosis after menopause; caffeine and alcohol can cause loss of calcium

Element *Minerals*	Need/Use	Where Found	Comments
Magnesium	Contributes to production of sex hormones	Meats, fish, dairy products, apples, apricots, nuts, seeds, leafy vegetables	Women suffering from PMS or menstrual cramps may get some relief from magnesium
Chromium	With insulin, is responsible for glucose utilization	Brewer's yeast, beer, clams, corn oil, wheat germ, chicken	Essential for someone with hypoglycemia
Selenium	Works with Vitamin E to reduce free radical damage in cells and protects the immune system	Brazil nuts, brown rice, whole milk, cottage cheese, garlic, eggs	Men need selenium since there is a high amount of it in semen

Element Minerals	Need/Use	Where Found	Comments
Iodine	Essential for functioning of thyroid gland and is an integral part of the hormone thyroxin, which controls many body aspects	Seafood, seaweed, onions, pineapple	Low levels can lead to a sluggish thyroid, irregular periods in women, or severe PMS
Manganese	Trace mineral important in activating many enzyme systems in body	Beets, nuts, whole grains, leafy green vegetables, apples, apricots	Required for utilization of thiamine, fatty acids, choline, and Vitamin C

As this chart suggests, there are many foods that can contribute to your sexual health and performance. All in all, remember that your sexual attitudes reflect your entire body's health. If you are malnourished, even on the smallest micro-level, you will have less interest in sex and romance, and your relations with your partner will suffer. But by eating properly—and taking ginseng—you will find that your sexual interest rejuvenates and flowers, making your intimate life much more satisfying and enjoyable.

▣ 5 ▣

Ginseng and Your Health

Good health and good sense are two of life's greatest blessings.

Publius Syrus, 42 B.C.

If there is one area in which ginseng has shown remarkable benefits outside of energizing your body, it is in improving your health. Since time immemorial, ginseng has had the reputation of being a potent tonic that restores a weak body to good health and maintains a healthy body in top shape. As mentioned earlier, traditional Chinese medicine has long considered ginseng to be the king of herbs, using it as the central ingredient in nearly every herbal mixture devised. Because of this reputation, many twentieth-century researchers have focused on understanding the science behind ginseng's ability to help people stay healthy and fight off disease more effectively than any other herbal remedy known.

To date, the research on ginseng has borne consistent results in this regard. It shows that, although ginseng does not cure any specific illness, it is effective in helping to prevent many types of diseases, particularly those that result from environmental, physical, or emotional stress to the body. This chapter will review the theoretical basis of disease and the stress–disease connection so that you can understand exactly how ginseng achieves its preventive effects. The chapter will then detail a number of specific diseases that ginseng has been shown to be effective against.

Ginseng and the Stress–Disease Connection

Modern science has made many strides in deepening our understanding of how diseases occur, but because the body's systems are so intricately interconnected and complex, much of our knowledge is still incomplete. The physiology and biochemistry of health and disease is especially complicated, but it is useful to explain some of the basics so that you can truly see how ginseng fits in.

First, let's define what is meant by health and disease. Obviously, good health is, in simple terms, the normal functioning of the entire human body, while disease is the breakdown or impairment of any of the body systems. Diseases can occur for many reasons and can cause problems of varying degrees. Most common diseases are created by the invasion of bacteria or viruses into the body, which cause infection and interrupt normal functioning. In most cases, the body's immune system can locate the infection and destroy the foreign cells. However, in some cases when the person is already weakened or has been overly taxed by the illness itself, the immune system does not function properly and the disease can infiltrate other parts of the body and cause secondary diseases.

Some diseases are noninfectious, but are created by environmental factors such as smoke, pollutants, and other chemicals that invade the body and trigger a malfunction. In these cases, the body struggles to regain its normal functioning, but the disease may continue to chronically affect the body over a long period of time so that it slowly deteriorates. Still other diseases, often called lifestyle diseases, are caused by wear and tear on the body due to improper or excessive eating, drinking, poor conditioning, or stress. These diseases can often be improved or cured by reversing the conditions that caused them, although in some cases, once the problem is triggered, such as with heart disease, it may never go away completely. Finally, some diseases, known as autoimmune diseases, are created by the body turning against itself and attacking normal cells. Autoimmune diseases include chronic fatigue syndrome and multiple sclerosis. Scientists do not yet understand most autoimmune diseases.

In this context, it now becomes clearer why ginseng has been shown to be especially effective against those diseases caused by stress. Stress wears the body down and depletes it of necessary nutrients, creates imbalances in many bodily systems, and ultimately weakens the immune system, opening the body up to invasion by a wide range of bacteria and viruses that can wreak havoc on the tissues of the body. You yourself have probably become ill on several occasions after hard physical labor, after being under pressure for long hours in order to meet a tight deadline, or after a family crisis that involved a lot of your attention and worry. These types of situations typically make us susceptible to diseases such as colds, influenza (flu), herpes, skin rashes, nausea, diarrhea, and high blood pressure. In some cases, medical researchers have also traced stress as a causative factor in a number of life-threatening diseases, such as diabetes, angina, certain types of cancers, and diseases of the immune system.

Ginseng is so effective in preventing stress-related illnesses because, as this book has pointed out, it bolsters the body's endocrine system, which plays a critical role in managing the body's response to stress of any kind. The active ingredients in ginseng, the ginsenosides or eleutherosides, directly support the body's hormonal system, and the benefits from this create a healthier organism that is better able to resist infections, diseases caused by general wear and tear, and perhaps certain diseases resulting from autoimmune dysfunction caused by stress.

It is worth noting that ginseng does not directly affect the body's immune system. Its active ingredients do not contribute chemicals to help hunt down and fight off infections, nor do they seem to strengthen the effects of the body's existing immune system cells that perform those killer operations. (However, ginseng does contain polysaccharides, large sugar-like molecules, that are believed to be immune system stimulants.) For the most part, however, ginseng does not cure a disease that has already struck. Instead, it works hand in hand with the body's endocrine system to keep it functioning in an efficient, healthy way so that the body can naturally resist disease before it strikes.

Of Health and Hormones

To better understand ginseng's role, let's now look at the body's amazing endocrine system in more depth. The endocrine system is extremely important in regu-

lating the many bodily functions that impact homeostasis, or the normal metabolic balance in the body.
This is because the glands of the endocrine system produce dozens of hormones that control our metabolism
and balance the levels of many critical chemicals in
the bloodstream, such as sodium, potassium, and calcium. The endocrine system is made up of a variety of
interlinked glands including:

- *the pituitary gland*—located at the base of the
  brain, the pituitary is the master gland that controls
  other endocrine glands; it also makes direct-acting
  hormones that affect the growth of the skeletal system, regulate the function of the thyroid gland, and
  affect the action of the gonads (testes and ovaries).
  The pituitary also produces substances that interact
  with the pancreas, as well as hormones that increase
  blood pressure and prevent excessive secretion of
  urine. In the 1970s, it was discovered that the pituitary also produces endorphins, the neuropeptides
  that increase our feelings of pleasure and reduce our
  sensitivity to pain.

- *the thyroid*—located in the front of the neck, the
  thyroid regulates the speed of most cellular reactions and the metabolic rate of the body, including
  oxygen consumption in the cells and energy consumption in the cells.

▣ *the parathyroids*—located adjacent to the thyroid
gland, the parathyroid glands produce hormones
that help control calcium and phosphate levels in
the blood.

▣ *the pancreas*—the pancreas affects digestion by releasing digestive juices into the intestines, but it is
also part of the endocrine system because it produces insulin, which affects the rate of sugar uti-
lization in cells and promotes the formation of
proteins and the storage of fat. The pancreas also
produces glucagon, which raises blood sugar levels
by releasing glucose from the liver.

▣ *the thymus*—located in the upper part of the
chest, the thymus plays a central role in establishing
the body's immunological capacities. The thymus
causes lymphocytes to become T-cells, which de-
fend against viruses and other infections.

▣ *the adrenal glands*—as discussed throughout this
book, the adrenals are involved in many bodily functions relating to the circulatory system, metabolism,
sexuality, and the body's response to acute stress. In
a quick review, the inner part of the adrenal glands
produce the hormones epinephrine (adrenaline)
and norepinephrine (noradrenaline) in response to
stimulation by the sympathetic nervous system
under arousal or stress. When stress occurs, these

hormones are central to the body's first response in preparation for fight or flight. They cause the blood vessels in the intestines, liver, and kidneys to constrict, and widen the blood vessels that feed the skeletal muscles. They also cause the heart rate to increase and the blood sugar to rise, giving the body more energy. Following that initial response, the outer part of the adrenal glands produce *glucocorticoid* hormones (such as cortisone and hydrocortisone) that help the body through the resistance phase of the three-phase stress response. The glucocorticoid hormones also help the body during periods of normal activity by stimulating the conversion of protein to energy and by controlling the concentration of salts and water in bodily fluids essential for the maintenance of life. They also influence the body's inflammatory reactions and to some extent the immune system. The hormones produced in the outer part of the adrenals are controlled by ACTH, produced in the pituitary gland in levels that vary according to your emotions, stress, or injury.

The glands of the endocrine system are intricately interconnected and, in several cases, the hormones produced by one gland provide "feedback" to another gland by provoking or inhibiting the production of other hormones. For example, when a certain amount of thyroid hormone is in the bloodstream, the pituitary stops releasing a thyroid-stimulating hormone, halting the production of more thyroid hormones. The glands are also highly sensitive to the metabolism and chemistry in the body. For instance, high levels of glucose in the blood stimulate the pancreas to produce insulin, while low blood sugar levels stimulate the adrenal gland to produce epinephrine and norepinephrine.

As you might imagine, with such a tightly connected system, any problem or malfunction in one gland can have vast repercussions on the entire endocrine system and on the body as a whole. This is precisely what happens under stress. Mild stress, such as that created by normal daily activity, causes the endocrine system to work hard, but the body can usually tolerate it without difficulty. However, difficult tasks such as acute physical exertion, prolonged mental exercise, or even ordinary activities undertaken when the body is tired, out of shape, or already weakened can be stressors of a more severe nature. When the body is taxed more than it can handle, your endocrine system is pushed to the limit, creating the potential for many types of malfunctions and problems that lead to lowered resistance and disease. For example, researchers know that when stress causes a prolongation in the production of corticosteroids, the adrenals become depleted, increasing the risk of diseases such as diabetes, high blood pressure, and cancer.

As you saw in Chapter 2, however, ginseng reduces the severity of many reactions in the endocrine system. It appears to alter the production of ACTH (produced by the pituitary gland) which in turn moderates the production of the adrenal hormones. Ginseng also seems to directly affect the adrenal glands, so that they react more quickly to stress and recover more quickly after producing their hormones. Again, it is also likely that these positive effects on the adrenal glands are passed on to the other endocrine glands, so that the whole system is healthier, more resilient, and stronger day in and day out.

Ginseng's Indirect Connection to the Immune System

Because the body's systems are so interlinked, it is also important to understand that improvements in one system tend to have beneficial effects in other systems. By virtue of its support of the endocrine system, ginseng creates other repercussions, especially in the brain and other nerve cells that produce neurotransmitters and neuropeptides, which control the immune system. In this way, one might say that ginseng actually does have an effect on the immune system, although it is indirect.

Here's how that connection occurs. Research has shown that when people are healthy and happy, the brain and nerve cells throughout the body produce fifty to sixty neuropeptides, such as those we call endorphins. Activities such as laughter, exercise, sex, and productive work and satisfying relationships tend to raise the level of endorphins in our body. These endorphins produce feelings of pleasure in the mind, but they also relax the muscles, release tension, and relieve pain. More importantly though, research has shown that a higher level of endorphins in the body creates a strengthened immune system. People who raise their endorphin levels literally have greater numbers of T-cells, N-cells, and gamma globulins, which are the cells that fight off bacteria and viruses as part of the immune response that continuously circulates in the bloodstream.

In contrast, and this is key, those people who have a great deal of stress generally exhibit significantly lower levels of endorphins in the body, indicating that stress either alters the production of endorphins and other neuropeptides or destroys them. This is why people who become stressed out or are depressed are often prone to a host of illnesses; without the endorphins to activate their immune systems, their bodies cannot fight off the viruses and bacteria that cause illness.

As you may guess, this is again where ginseng fits in. Because ginseng, by supporting the hormonal system, allows the body to moderate the stress response, the body is less taxed and thus more capable of producing—or at least not destroying—the endorphins and other neuropeptides that strengthen the immune system. In other words, by keeping the endocrine system in shape, ginseng gives the body a chance to use its natural endorphins to spur the immune system into action. While no direct research has yet been done to prove this, several experiments seem to confirm this hypothesis. In one double-blind study, thirty-six healthy subjects received either ten milliliters of a Siberian ginseng fluid or a placebo on a daily basis for four weeks. The group that received the ginseng demonstrated significant improvements in a variety of immune system parameters. Most notable were a significant increase in T-helper cells and an increase in natural killer cell activity. In another study, performed in Europe, three groups of twenty subjects were given either a capsule with 100 mg of aqueous ginseng, a capsule of lactose, or a capsule containing a standardized ginseng extract (G115). All three groups took the capsules for eight weeks. Blood samples were taken at the beginning of the study, at the end of four weeks, and at the end of the eight weeks. The results indicated that at the end of the eight weeks, the group that had taken the standardized ginseng extract had significantly higher levels of total lymphocytes, T-helper cells, and suppressor cells than the placebo group given lactose. Meanwhile, there has also been research in India that indicates that ginseng also may help the body in this indirect manner to produce more interferon, an antiviral protective protein.

Taking Ginseng to Counter a Range of Diseases and Ailments

With this explanation of how ginseng works, let's now examine the many health benefits that ginseng seems to bring. Here are a few of the diseases and illnesses that ginseng seems to help the most.

Colds, Flu, and Generalized Illness

Ginseng seems to help the body to resist many types of low-level illnesses that commonly strike the body under stress, such as colds and flu. For example, in one study conducted by Itskovity Brekhman, drivers of heavy trucks took Siberian ginseng extract in their tea for a period of six years. Over the course of the treatment, the number of drivers who became ill from influenza dropped from forty-one per thousand to less than three per thousand. The number of days lost per year to sickness dropped from 286 per 100 workers to 11. In another long-term study, more than 60,000 Soviet workers in a car manufacturing factory in Togliatti were given a daily dose of Siberian ginseng for several months. Their general health improved, and the number of absentee days due to general illness was sharply reduced.

I have recommended ginseng to many of my patients, and the majority report that, thanks to the ginseng, they stop getting low-level illnesses such as colds, fevers, headaches, and the like. As Eric Harr, the triathlete you met in Chapter 3, told me, even when you put your body under great duress (like training for the Olympics), your ability to resist disease greatly expands when you take ginseng. Harr reported that since taking ginseng, he had not been sick once.

Healing and Inflammations

Because the hormones produced by glands in the endocrine system regulate blood pressure and the chemical nature (e.g., the levels of sodium, potassium, and calcium) of the blood, the improvements caused by ginseng in the endocrine system appear to also have an effect on the ability of the body to heal bruises and fight inflammations. These effects have been proven in studies carried out by Soviet and Japanese researchers.

Digestive Ailments

Many common illnesses are related to digestion. In this regard, research has supported the use of ginseng to improve digestion. Some studies on animals also show that ginseng increases the rate of RNA synthesis in liver cells, thus improving their functioning. Increased RNA synthesis also has a positive effect on the digestive system. Other studies show that ginseng elevates plasma HDL (good cholesterol) while lowering LDL (bad cholesterol) levels.

High Blood Pressure

Studies have shown that ginseng is useful in normalizing blood pressure, whether it is too high or too low. In one study, a group of 540 volunteers suffering from hypertension showed significant improvement in normalizing blood pressure when given ginseng. A variety of studies on elderly people with high blood pressure showed that ginseng lowered it modestly. The effects of ginseng seem to be especially significant when used in combination with a comprehensive program that includes dietary changes, exercise, and the learning of relaxation techniques. In China, ginseng is used in hospitals to raise blood pressure as part of emergency treatment after shock, loss of blood, or a heart attack.

Diabetes

In a healthy individual the pancreas produces the hormone insulin, which facilitates the entry of glucose into the cells of the body, where it is consumed for energy. In a person with diabetes, however, either the pancreas produces too little insulin, or the insulin produced does not activate the receptors in the body's cells to let the glucose in. As a result, people with diabetes end up with an excessive buildup of sugar in their bloodstream and urine. In acute cases, especially in the case of people born with the disease, diabetes can lead to coma and even death, because the body does not get energy from the sugar in cells and so breaks down stored fat. This produces compounds in the blood called *ketone bodies*, which make the blood acidic and interfere with respiration. In chronic situations, especially among overweight adults who develop diabetes at midlife, the moderately high sugar levels in their blood can lead to a number of problems, including kidney disease, loss of sight due to rupturing of the blood vessels in the eyes, and numbness in the limbs due to a reduction in the blood flow. Diabetics also have an increased risk of heart attack and stroke, and diabetic women who become pregnant have an increased incidence of stillbirths and birth defects.

There are typically two treatments to help diabetics control their blood sugar levels. In Type I diabetes (which refers to people who develop diabetes as children, usually because their pancreas does not function properly), the standard treatment is to administer insulin injections to supplement the body's low levels of insulin. In Type II diabetes (which refers to diabetes caused by ineffective insulin, often found in overweight adults), the treatment usually consists of a significant change in diet to avoid overwhelming the body with blood sugar after meals. This means that Type II diabetics generally must not consume foods that contain the simple forms of sugar (glucose, fructose, lactose) in large quantities, eating instead polysaccharides, which are broken down slowly in the stomach before being released as sugar into the bloodstream.

Although it is not yet clear why, ginseng has been shown to improve both types of diabetes. Ginseng appears to help bolster the body against the stress of continual insulin injections. Like any invasive procedure, injections subject the body to a harsh challenge, but ginseng seems to help the hormonal system rebalance itself quickly. Because of its adaptogenic properties, ginseng also helps normalize the blood sugar level, raising or lowering it as the body requires. In one series of experiments on healthy humans who were given 100 g of sugar water, those whose sugar water included 2 ml of ginseng did not undergo a rise in blood sugar level during the first hour, as did the control group. By the end of the third hour, the blood sugar level in the ginseng group fell to 23% below its initial level. In many experiments on animals, again, those animals who had received an extract of ginseng had lower blood sugar levels than animals in the control group.

Anemia

Traditional Chinese medicine has long used ginseng to treat anemia, and now several modern experiments appear to confirm the wisdom of this tradition. In one study, fifty patients who had not had success with other antianemia medications were treated with ginseng. Their red blood cell counts rose, and they also experienced a decrease in several subjective symptoms, such as fatigue.

Chronic Fatigue Syndrome and Generalized Fatigue

Ginseng has been shown to exert a number of beneficial effects that may be useful in the treatment of both chronic fatigue syndrome and generalized fatigue. In regard to the latter, because ginseng improves the body's general health and ability to combat stress, the body ends up with more energy and vitality. I have used ginseng in this capacity for many of my patients. In one case, a sixty-eight-year-old woman came to me because she was constantly exhausted. For almost three months she had been feeling tired and unable to accomplish much during the day. I prescribed two capsules of 500 mg extract of Siberian ginseng (equivalent to five grams of ginseng root) and within two days, she told me that she felt a powerful renewal of her energy. She began rising early in the morning and attending to her affairs as she had not done in the previous three months. What was most astonishing about this case is that she had tried many other remedies, to no avail. Ginseng was the only product that renewed her energy to a level where she could function normally again.

Chronic fatigue syndrome (CFS), however, is a specific disease state in which people become abnormally exhausted after even the briefest activities. Their energy becomes quickly depleted, and they are seldom able to sustain effort or concentration for very long. Other symptoms of CFS include a recurrent sore throat, low-grade fevers, lymph node swelling, muscle and joint pain, intestinal discomfort, emotional distress, depression, and loss of concentration. While many people originally doubted that CFS was a legitimate disease, it has now been officially recognized by the Center for Disease Control in the United States and by many other health organizations in countries around the world. Some researchers believe that the causes of CFS are related to the Epstein-Barr virus, which is a member of the herpes group of viruses. Other researchers have proposed a number of other viruses as the cause of CFS. Most of the proposed viral agents are of the sort that establish lifelong latent infection opportunities. Such viruses remain in the body in latent form and are kept in check by a healthy immune system. However, as soon as the immune system is run down, the virus strikes.

People with these types of viruses are subject to infection many times over the course of their life. Blood samples from patients with CFS confirm this; the samples reveal lower levels of natural killer (NK) cells and reduced levels of lymphocytes, key white blood cells that battle viruses. It has also been noted that CFS patients have lower levels of interferon, a special chemical factor produced by the body as a natural protector against viruses.

Again, because ginseng helps to strengthen the body's response to stress and indirectly supports the immune system, it has become highly regarded as a potential ally in combating CFS. In general, research supports the fact that ginseng improves certain aspects of the illness. In one study conducted at the University of Buenos Aires in Argentina with fifty patients, researchers identified the following attributes of CFS: reduced mental alertness, emotional liability, lack of motivation and initiative, irritability, hostility, indifference to surroundings, unsociability, uncooperative behavior, lack of personal care and hygiene, and lack of appetite. The patients were first given a placebo pill for two weeks and then tested on several measures of mental acuity and attention. They were then given a standardized ginseng extract (G115), following which the tests were repeated. The researchers found that the administration of ginseng for the fifty-six days caused a substantial improvement in many areas, especially in the patients' attention and concentration.

Heart Disease

Stress is a significant factor in heart disease, so by virtue of its ability to help the body reduce stress, ginseng has often been correlated with reducing heart disease. In fact, many studies show that ginseng enhances blood circulation, normalization of blood pressure, reduction of cholesterol levels, and favorable shifts in protein and lipid metabolism. In one study, 206 patients were treated with ginseng; 75% showed a reduction of cholesterol levels, and 62% showed a reduction in high blood pressure.

In another study, Chinese red ginseng was tested on patients with serious congestive heart failure. The patients were divided into three groups: the first group was given red ginseng; the second group received dioxin, a cardiac stimulant derived from the digitalis plant and long used on heart patients; and the third group received a combination of the two. The patients in the second and third groups showed the best improvement on a number of measures.

Researchers in China have given purified ginseng ginsenosides to patients after open heart surgery. In comparison to patients not given this compound, those given ginsenosides experienced better recovery and less tissue damage.

Menopause

Ginseng seems to assist women in dealing with menopause. In one clinical study, eighty-three patients took ginseng over a period of eight weeks. Symptoms such as hot flashes, weakness, and fatigue were reduced in seventy of the test subjects.

Surgery and Recovery

Surgery is very debilitating to the body, producing a high level of stress on many bodily systems. In fact, the amount of time it takes for people to recover from surgery has been shown to be highly linked to the stress caused by the operation. Given this debilitating nature of surgery, a number of studies have been conducted using ginseng on people undergoing surgery. In one study involving 120 postoperative gynecological patients, 60 were given ginseng on a daily basis while 60 received a placebo. The patients who were given ginseng experienced significant increases in their levels of hemoglobin, protein, and hematocrit (percentage of red blood cells in total volume of blood), as well as body weight, all of which are important measures of recovery. In a Korean study as well, surgery patients who received ginseng recovered more quickly.

Dr. David Morrow, a board-certified cosmetic surgeon, dermatologist, and founder of the Morrow Institute for Specialty Plastic Surgery in Rancho Mirage, California, has started to give ginseng to his patients in order to boost their immune systems and assist in their speedy recovery. His patients begin taking ginseng a few days before the surgery and continue with it for two weeks afterward. He reports that he has noticed a definite improvement in the recovery rates of his patients, and he points out that many of his patients are so pleased by the overall energizing and healthful benefits of ginseng that they continue to take it for months afterward on their own.

In one of my most difficult cases, I had as a patient a six-year-old girl suffering from leukemia. She had been undergoing chemotherapy, which had made her extremely sick. At the time, my office was on the second floor of a building and this girl had difficulty even climbing the steps to see me. Her father was a medical doctor, and to my surprise he was willing to let me prescribe Siberian ginseng for her. Within one month, the ginseng had reinvigorated her and reduced her nausea from the chemotherapy treatments. To my delight, she began having no problems climbing the steps to my office, and she was soon doing many things that normal six-year-olds do. This girl has now fully recovered from the leukemia, and I am confident that the ginseng helped her tolerate the doses of chemotherapy that she was forced to undergo to save her life.

Cancer and Radiation Treatments

A number of statistical studies have been conducted to assess the effectiveness of ginseng in preventing certain types of cancers. In one study, nearly two thousand pairs of volunteers were divided into two groups. One group had been diagnosed with various cancers, while those in the other group were healthy. The statisticians determined that ginseng users had a lower risk of cancers of the lip, oral cavity, pharynx, esophagus, stomach, colon, rectum, liver, pancreas, larynx, lungs, and ovaries. In addition, even smokers who had taken ginseng regularly had a lower risk of cancer. However, there was no improvement in the risk factors for cancers of the breast, uterus, cervix, urinary bladder, and thyroid gland. In a follow-up study, the same researchers compared two groups of nine hundred-plus subjects and found the same lower incidence of cancer among the ginseng users. However, it has been noted that the researchers did not take into account dietary factors and other health habits. Critics have suggested that those who took the time to take ginseng may simply have had better health habits in general. Nevertheless, the results of these two studies are quite intriguing.

In addition, ginseng has been shown to be very effective in reducing the deleterious effects of radiation exposure, such as that received by cancer patients. Ginseng seems to help return both white and red blood cell counts to normal after radiation treatment has lowered them. In fact, ginseng is commonly used in China as an adjunct to both chemotherapy and radiation therapy. Chinese researchers report that the combination of ginseng usage and either chemotherapy or radiation therapy has raised the survival rates of cancer patients.

It is also theorized that ginseng helps the patient withstand the stress of these treatments; chemotherapy and radiation therapy are both extremely taxing on the body. Many patients are so taxed that they develop secondary cancers. In Korea, ginseng was shown to help patients tolerate cancer treatment, with fewer side effects such as nausea and fatigue. At the prestigious Soviet cancer facility, the Petrov Oncological Institute, it was found that one teaspoonful of concentrated Siberian ginseng enabled patients to take 50% more of anticancer drugs, and the patients lived longer as a result.

HIV Patients

There is a growing body of anecdotal evidence that supports the use of Siberian ginseng as a complement to the use of drugs in the treatment of HIV patients. Over the past decade I have recommended Siberian ginseng to hundreds of HIV patients that I have treated. One patient was diagnosed with HIV in the early 1980s, and has been taking Siberian ginseng since 1988. At the time of this writing, he was still doing well, having been able to fend off full-blown AIDS for more than a decade. For the past few years, I have attended many professional workshops such as The HIV, AIDS, and Chinese Medicine Conference. Many practitioners have shared the favorable results they have had using ginseng and Chinese herbal medicine in the treatment of HIV-related symptomatology.

Depression, Insomnia, and Mood Problems

Ginseng has also been shown to help with a range of emotional illnesses and mood problems. In one experiment, fifty men and women with depression between the ages of twenty-four and sixty-six were tested on a variety of intellectual and cognitive functions. They were then given two capsules of a standardized ginseng concentrate each day for fifty-six days. Following this period of ginseng usage, they were again given the same tests and their respective scores were compared. The mean scores for all patients on certain of the items, such as information comprehension, visual comprehension, observation, and practical reasoning improved in a statistically significant way. There were also improvements in several measures of emotional balance, such as motivation, incentive, cooperation, and personal care.

Ginseng appears to simply make people feel better, as if they are more in control of their lives. In an experiment that was conducted at a high-technology company in Stockholm, Sweden, 390 test subjects were divided into two groups: one received ginseng, the other a placebo. By the end of the study, which lasted twelve weeks, those subjects who were taking ginseng were tested and measured to have a better appetite, higher levels of alertness, and they were more relaxed. Dubbed "quality of life," this study especially reinforced that people who had the lowest scores at the outset were the ones who benefited the most from taking ginseng. In another study of ninety-five middle managers in an English manufacturing company, similar results were obtained between the ginseng and placebo groups. In this experiment, those managers who took a combination vitamin/mineral/ginseng capsule versus a placebo were evaluated as having greater improvement in the subscales of tension and anxiety reduction and mood, especially in those subjects who were rated as having a poor diet to begin with. While the study was too small to draw firm conclusions, the researchers felt that the results were a valid indication that quality of life improves with ginseng.

Your Own Total Care Program

Without a doubt, we are fortunate to be living today. For the past several decades, doctors and medical researchers have learned more and more about how we can improve our health so that we can be happier, more fit, and live longer. In the last twenty years alone, the average life span for a man has increased from seventy to seventy-two, and for a woman from seventy-seven to seventy-eight. However, stress continues to be among the most common causes of illness and disease.

Stress may also be a factor in two of the three most common causes of death in the United States: heart disease and cancer.

Ultimately, as this chapter has shown, whatever you can do to lower your stress reaction can go a long way toward improving your health and lengthening your life. In this regard, the major benefit of adding ginseng to your diet is that it reduces stress, which in turn improves your health and builds your resistance to many types of diseases. If, like many of my patients and others I know, you begin taking ginseng on a regular basis, you too will begin to feel stronger and more physically fit, and you will notice that your resistance to disease improves.

Ginseng, Aging, and Longevity

Nothing makes one old so quickly as the ever present thought that one is growing older . . .

G. C. Lichtenberg
(1742–1799),
German physicist,
philosopher

Considering that ginseng reduces the harmful effects of stress chemicals in your body, enhances your metabolism and circulation, and guards against many types of disease, it should come as no surprise that ginseng can add years to your life. The logic of this is obvious: when you are less stressed, in better shape, and have fewer illnesses, you are much more likely to stay healthy and live longer.

However, since the biology of human aging and the factors that determine longevity are enormously complex, it is clearly worthwhile to understand in more detail about how ginseng affects longevity. This chapter will therefore present what scientists now understand about how and why we age, and where in this equation ginseng fits.

Will You Still Need Me When I'm Sixty-Four?

The famous Beatles' song about getting old by age sixty-four was really never accurate. Over the course of the last several centuries, the average human life span has increased tremendously, more than tripling since the 1700s alone. In 1796, the average human life span was just twenty-five years, by 1896 it was forty-eight years, and by 1996 it had increased to almost eighty years (for people in developed countries). For many people, being sixty-four is almost like being a spring chicken; they still have plenty of verve and vitality left in them, and their lives in retirement only get more exciting. Some scientists project that the human life span will rise to 120 or even 150 by the year 2050. Scientists even expect that they will eventually discover ways to help people live for several hundred years!

But the good news about increasing life span is not just that science is helping people live to a later age, but that researchers are discovering the keys to helping people stay younger and healthier for decades longer. After all, there is little value in living an extra thirty to fifty years if you are weak, debilitated, and unable to perform the normal activities of life. Most of us naturally want to live our senior years as energetically and actively as our younger years, and want to be free of disease and infirmity so we can enjoy the blessings of retirement. When researchers today talk about prolonging life, they are talking about ways to slow or halt the aging process in order to prolong youth.

In this sense, the antiaging field encompasses two approaches:

▣ learning how to slow or halt *normal* aging that occurs via the slow degeneration of the body over time, including wrinkles, reduced muscular strength and mobility, cataracts and poor vision, loss of bone mass, etc;

▣ learning how to prevent the *pathologic* aging caused by hereditary or lifestyle diseases such as diabetes and arthritis, which may later bring on cardiovascular disease or osteoporosis.

Both tasks are necessary to fulfill in order to reach the goal of living to 120 or 150 without becoming chronically sick, decrepit, or incapacitated by disease.

Unfortunately, the specifics of why humans age are still not very clear to scientists, and so the discovery of comprehensive solutions to counter the two types of aging remains elusive. In recent years though, scientists have originated many new ideas and developed a number of theories about aging that seem to make a great deal of sense. More importantly, nearly every one of these theories has led researchers to at least one useful discovery that is at least partially effective in staving off either normal or pathologic aging. As a result, there is now a tremendous amount of excitement in medicine that we will very soon fully uncover the secrets to greater health and a significantly longer life span for us all.

The Theories of Aging

In general, scientists believe that aging is a natural part of evolution. The evolutionary rationale for aging is that we are no longer "needed" once we have produced children during our period of greatest sexual fertility and have passed on our wisdom to them. This premise fits in with most of the history of human life; men and women have usually had children by at least the age of twenty and have died by the age of forty. As harsh as it sounds, the constant turnover of people over eons of time has allowed for the reproduction of the species while preserving the resources needed to feed them.

In the animal kingdom, aging does not occur to the same degree as it does in humans. Animals do not seem to age as distinctly as humans and generally die as a result of natural causes. This has led scientists to wonder how and why the process of biological aging came to support the evolutionary need.

In answer to this question, there are two broad groups of theories. The first is that aging is programmed into our genes, like other evolutionary traits of *Homo sapiens* that are passed down through our DNA. This theory proposes that our body has a sort of biological clock that essentially ticks down the years and knows when to set the aging process in motion. This is first seen when the clock sets into motion the process of sexual maturation as we go from childhood to young adulthood. Continued aging from adulthood to death is thus simply the continuation of that process.

In contrast, the other main group of theories about aging is focused on the idea that the physical manifestations of growing old occur accidentally and randomly. The premise in these theories is that while nature intended us to die after we procreate, it left it to chance how and when this would occur. As a result, our body is susceptible to various forces that create "errors" in our metabolism, making us prone to disease and decay.

To understand where ginseng fits into all this, let's look in more depth at a few of the theories of aging within each group. The following section presents briefly the fundamental concepts of five leading contenders, including why some scientists believe in each theory and why others don't. Once we review all of these ideas, we'll explain how the pharmacology of ginseng responds to every hypothesis. In this way, you'll see how, whichever theory turns out to be correct (or even if several do), ginseng can be a significant part of your own antiaging program.

Aging by Accident

Let's begin with the group of theories that proposes that aging occurs through random and accidental quirks that slowly bring about the physical manifestations of age.

The "Wear and Tear" Theory

The "wear and tear" theory proposes that the body and its cells are damaged by normal use and abuse over time. The organs of the body (particularly the liver, stomach, kidneys, and skin) are susceptible to stress and toxins from our diet and the environment, which wear them down each passing year. The consumption of foods such as fats, sugars, caffeine, and alcohol constitute abuses that especially tax the organs, but even the normal day-to-day activities of life that expose us to the sun's rays and force us to use our bodies are also inevitable causes of wear and tear. In short, the process of life itself creates aging, and not much can be done to prevent this.

In this theory, the actual cause of aging is not simply the wear and tear, but that, as we grow older, the body cannot repair itself fast enough to counteract the problems created by this use and abuse. When we are young, our bodies produce enough of the necessary chemicals to combat toxins in the body, and they work efficiently at fixing cellular wear and tear. However, as we age, the body loses this ability to repair and maintain its systems quickly, so more cells are worn and torn before the body can replace them. Thus, we both age and become more prone to infirmities and diseases.

There is clearly a certain amount of logic to the "wear and tear" theory; it makes sense that no organism can go on forever in perfect operating condition. The idea of excessive wear and tear being caused by abuse, such as a poor diet, excessive drinking, smoking, or exposure to environmental toxins seems especially valid. After all, we cannot expect the cells in a body to function normally and indefinitely if they are poisoned or forced to work in unnatural conditions.

Critics of this theory maintain that it does not go deep enough in explaining what causes the phenomenon to happen, nor does it completely cover why aging occurs. In response, one scientist has proposed that wear and tear may directly affect the power plants in cells, the *mitochondria*, that provide energy for all the cells' activities. With wear and tear, the mitochondria become damaged and cannot repair themselves. Since they contain a piece of DNA that gives instructions for the manufacture of cellular proteins, damaged mitochondria cause the cells to function improperly, initiating the aging process.

The Free Radical Theory

The free radical approach to aging takes the wear and tear theory one step further in trying to explain more precisely how the body deteriorates. The term *free radical* describes any molecule in the body that differs from normal molecules by virtue of possessing a free electron. In a normal molecule, the electrons are paired, so the electrical charge is balanced, but in a free radical molecule, the extra electron causes an unstable state, and the molecule has a negative charge. As a result, it looks to "steal" an electron from normal molecules, but in so doing, it creates a new free radical, and the process continues.

The problem with free radicals, it is believed, is that they upset the harmony of the body. Free radicals are thought to attack cell membranes and in the process produce waste products that are toxic to our cells because they destroy or disturb the normal DNA and RNA synthesis occuring within the cells. It is also thought that free radicals interfere with the synthesis of protein and thus lower the amount of energy available to you and prevent the body from building muscle mass. Free radicals also destroy enzymes needed for vital chemical processes in the metabolism. Not only do free radicals thus promote aging, but they are also associated as a causative factor in heart disease, cancers, skin problems, and autoimmune diseases.

Many scientists use the term *oxidation* to refer to the destructive nature of free radicals in the body. Just as rust forms from adding oxygen to metals, free radicals form when certain cells encounter oxygen, which causes the loss of an electron within the cell. In fact, one proof that scientists have used to demonstrate the validity of the free radical theory is that certain chemicals, called antioxidants, inhibit the formation of free radicals and seem to prevent aging. Chief among these antioxidants are the vitamins C, E, and beta-carotene, which the body converts to vitamin A. These vitamins prevent oxygen from producing free radicals, as many experiments with animals have proven.

The free radical theory has become one of the most highly intriguing as well as one of the most accepted of the theories of aging. Nevertheless, some critics argue that it does not fully explain aging because in many experiments on free radicals, the lab animals that were given high doses of antioxidants have also eaten less food. These critics contend that because antioxidants taste bad, the experimental animals are repelled from eating. The critics charge that the reduced diet slows down the metabolism, which then slows down the aging process, and so the experiments don't prove that the antioxidants and the free radicals are truly implicated as the cause of aging. Nevertheless, this theory has much support these days and is being studied in many other experiments.

The Immune System Theory

The immune system theory holds that over time the immune system stops functioning in its normal fashion as the body's line of defense against foreign substances that enter the body and interfere with the proper functioning of cells. The theory rests on two major findings: first, that with age, the level of antibodies in the body declines; and second, that many autoimmune diseases occur with age, indicating that the body loses its ability to distinguish between its own cells and foreign cells.

Critics of this theory hold that the immune system is affected by many other things in the body, such as hormones and the nervous system, so the theory does not truly get to the source of the aging problem. It may be that there is a more basic reason to explain why the immune system breaks down.

Aging by the Clock

Let's now look at the leading theories that contend that there is a biological clock that controls aging.

The Neuroendocrine Theory

The neuroendocrine theory holds that the body's hormonal system, led by the hypothalamus, is responsible for determining aging. The hypothalamus regulates the endocrine glands in the body, which in turn control many critical processes, including growth, metabolism, energy production, cellular repair—and sexual maturity. As we age and reach the point of sexual maturity, our body knows that it has reached its evolutionary goal to propagate the species. Beyond that point, there is no true reason to maintain the same level of hormonal upkeep, so according to this theory, the hypothalamus begins to produce less and less of its hormones and the entire endocrine system slowly ceases to function properly. A chain reaction then occurs: the metabolism slows down, our ability to produce energy declines, and our immune systems become weakened.

Recent research has also uncovered a hormone, dubbed DHEA (dehydroepiandrosterone), which is produced by the adrenal glands and seems to control the production of the other adrenal hormones, including corticosteroids, testosterone, estrogen, and progesterone. In this research, it was learned that DHEA production is very high in infants and remains so until a person is about twenty-five years old, and then begins to decline sharply. By the time we are sixty-five, we produce only 10% to 20% of the amount of DHEA we produced when we were twenty years old. This falling off of the hormone has led scientists to correlate the production of DHEA directly with aging. And since the hypothalamus controls the adrenal glands, it is believed that the whole process is biologically determined by the clock in the hypothalamus.

Proof for this theory has been demonstrated in many types of experiments, on both animals and humans. For example, in experiments with older mice, injections of DHEA caused the animals to renew their production of antibodies to levels equal to young mice. One researcher has also reported that DHEA injections stimulated production of T-cells, which fight off foreign invaders in cells. Other experiments have shown that DHEA improves the immune system and helps animals recover more quickly from disease. Several studies have shown that DHEA fends off cancer that has been injected in animals, including mammary tumors (breast cancer), prostate cancer, and other tumors. In addition, human studies have shown that DHEA levels are low in people with Alzheimer's disease and diabetes, in men with myocardial infarction (heart disease), and in women with osteoporosis.

Further proof for the hormonal theory of aging is that when people are given synthetic or animal hormone treatments, they rejuvenate and sometimes age more slowly. For example, adrenal extracts made from beef have been used since the 1930s to combat allergies and inflammations.

The critics of this theory contend that, as with the immune system theory, holding any one bodily system responsible for aging is an oversimplification. Some experiments have also been criticized for the same reasons as those experiments involving antioxidants and free radicals: when the lab animals receive DHEA injections they eat less, and thus it may be their slower metabolisms that are really responsible for the antiaging effects. Nevertheless, supporters of this theory contend that the hormonal system influences the body in many critical ways, from metabolism to immunity, and so it is very possible that our biological clock truly runs our hormonal system and determines our life span.

The Genetic Control Theory

The other major theory under scrutiny today, the genetic control theory, holds that our DNA is encoded with a preprogrammed set of instructions that determines how quickly we age and how long we live. However, because we are all unique individuals, there is some variation in our programs, which is why some people live to age seventy-five and others to one hundred. Evidence for this theory is quite profound; just as our DNA is programmed to turn us into humans when a sperm meets an egg at the moment of our conception, it is equally programmed to determine the remaining chronology of our lives. In fact, it is widely accepted in science that when DNA programs our embryonic formation, it already includes the concept of "cell death," which can be seen when cells die away from the mass of tissue that forms our hands, leaving spaces between our fingers. Since cell death already exists, claim the proponents of this theory, it is likely that our DNA is also programmed to create cell death as we age.

There are many critics of this theory who believe that it is flawed in many ways. For example, it fails to explain why we have been able to increase our life span so significantly. Our original DNA obviously could not have "known" that modern science would be able to preserve people till the age of 80 or even 120.

Ginseng and Aging Theories

There are many other theories of aging in addition to the five listed above. However, most of them are variations of one of the preceding theories, speculating either that an abundance of toxins or waste products in our cells create malfunctions that lead to aging and death, or that the body is somehow programmed to malfunction in such a way as to allow aging to occur.

Whichever hypothesis you subscribe to, however, the good news is that ginseng can help retard aging because of its innate chemical and pharmacological properties that counteract most suspected causes. Here's how:

The "Wear and Tear" Theory

Ginseng reduces wear and tear on the body because it lessens the chemical effects of stress; increases your ability to use oxygen in your muscle tissue, which gives you greater stamina and endurance; and indirectly supports your immune system against disease. As you may recall from Chapter 2, it is also thought that ginseng has a beneficial effect on the mitochondria in cells, increasing their ability to produce energy. Overall, this means that your body is less prone to wear and tear, thus effectively slowing down the aging process.

Much anecdotal evidence exists to support ginseng as a general antidote to wear and tear. The best evidence are the millions of people in China and in other parts of the world who have taken ginseng their entire lives, many of whom appear to be younger and healthier than their chronological counterparts who have not taken ginseng. Clearly, this is a difficult comparison to make, since so many factors influence how old a person looks and feels, and how long he or she lives. Nevertheless, people who take ginseng over long periods of time swear they feel younger and healthier than they would have if they had not taken ginseng.

The Free Radical Theory

The chemistry of ginseng fits in extremely well with the free radical theory of aging because, as you have seen, ginseng has been shown to significantly aid in improving the body's metabolism and use of oxygen. By stimulating the body's metabolism, ginseng reduces the dysfunctions that allow for the formation of free radicals. Another possible aid that ginseng provides is that it improves the ability of the liver to eliminate fatty lipids and lower LDL cholesterol, both of which seem to be key elements in the production of free radicals.

Research on reduced calorie diets suggests that high levels of glucose in the bloodstream impair or deactivate enzymes, proteins, and even the DNA in our genes. It is thought that this process contributes to the making of free radicals. Since ginseng helps regulate the level of glucose in the blood, this may be another benefit it offers to counteract the aging forces of free radicals.

The Immune System Theory

Ginseng fits into the immune system theory in an obvious way. As you learned in Chapter 5, ginseng's effect on the hormonal system plays an important part in assisting the immune system in several ways. First, because ginseng strengthens the adrenals and helps the body moderate its stress response by reducing the amount of corticosteroids in your blood, your immune system is less taxed. Like a car that is driven only five thousand miles a year instead of twenty thousand, your immune system thus has the ability to last longer and work better for many years. In addition, ginseng beneficially affects the hormonal system, which in turn stimulates the neurotransmitters that ultimately strengthen the immune system and make it more responsive to foreign agents.

The Neuroendocrine Theory

If you accept the neuroendocrine theory, ginseng has perhaps its strongest appeal as a rejuvenator, given that its most noted and proven effects on the body deal with improving the adrenal glands and perhaps the entire endocrine system. Of course, the problem is that this theory purports that the hypothalamus is preprogrammed to initiate aging according to a biological clock; you may wonder how ginseng can counteract the force of evolution. The answer is that while ginseng cannot ultimately prevent death, it can at least bolster the hormonal system to slow the aging process and make the body more resistant to disease. In fact, as mentioned earlier, there is extensive research that suggests that DHEA, produced in the adrenal glands, is a key element in preventing heart disease, Alzheimer's disease, diabetes, and many types of cancers.

The Genetic Control Theory

The genetic theory is the most difficult to counter in any way, whether one is touting more exercise, vitamin C, or ginseng as the key to longevity. If our genetics is so tightly programmed that, barring accidents, the day of our death is already predicted in our genetic code, then nothing will help us. However, this scenario seems quite inconsistent with the evidence of evolution, so if genetics plays a role in longevity, it is likely to be a much less predictable one. If that is so, ginseng does indeed offer some hope for increased longevity because, as indicated previously, it may prevent the apparent natural damage that occurs in our DNA over time. Given that ginseng helps the body burn oxygen and glucose more efficiently, and helps reduce the quantity of toxins, waste products, and perhaps free radicals in the bloodstream, it is very conceivable that it can play a role in slowing the clock that tells the DNA you are ready to get old.

Some Provocative Experiments

Unfortunately, there have been few long-term studies to validate ginseng's role in directly increasing longevity. However, there are a few studies that are interesting to note:

- In one study with animals conducted by Itskovity Brekhman, ginseng was given to rats in their drinking water every other day for 320 days. Treated animals lived an average of 799 days, versus 659 days for those animals that were not given ginseng.

- In another study, 358 patients between the ages of fifty and eighty-five were given a sugar-coated tablet of purified ginseng three times daily for two months while 123 patients were given a placebo. The researchers reported that the group given ginseng experienced significant improvements in memory and an increase in white blood cells and in the effectiveness of other immune functions. Also, the ginsenosides appeared to relieve symptoms of angina pectoris and heart irregularities.

▣ In a double-blind study that lasted for sixty days, ninety-eight patients between the ages of fifty and seventy were given either a ginseng extract mixed with vitamins and minerals or a placebo. The goal of this experiment was to determine the overall effect of the mixture, which was intended to be sold as a "geriatric ginseng." At the end of the test, the group given ginseng had significant improvement in many parameters, including fatigue, level of activity, initiative, and intellectual drive.

▣ In another study, forty-nine patients were given a similar "geriatric ginseng" mixture containing ginseng plus vitamins and minerals for four weeks, while another group of forty-nine were given a placebo. At the end of this experiment, the patients who were given ginseng had substantial improvements in alleviating depression, tension, insomnia, concentration, muscle fatigue, and in reinvigorating the subject's interest in life.

Such experiments largely validate the conclusions that many other experiments have made about the overall enhancing effects of ginseng on mental and physical performance regardless of the age of the subjects. Although these conclusions may seem to be too general to relate to longevity, they do at least support the fact that if you are going to live longer, you can do so in better health. For this reason alone, they are indicative of how ginseng can help you as you age.

The Long War

Given the fact that each of us is unique, it is likely that no single solution may work for all people in the effort to combat aging. It may very well be that each of the theories previously cited holds some degree of truth; thus, it may ultimately be futile to try to discover a way to completely avoid aging and death. Inevitably, the forces of evolution will simply win out, no matter what we do.

In my personal opinion, aging likely happens because of a combination of factors, including the biological clock that ticks away and eventually winds down, and the wear and tear that is caused by our lifestyle and worsened by chemical dysfunctions or imbalances that are created by toxins we ingest or encounter in the environment. The way I see it working is as follows: our biological clocks may actually allow us to live until 120 or even 150, but this generous life span is shortened by the strain we put on our body, the pace at which we wear it down, and/or the number of elements we encounter, such as stress, toxins, and free radicals, all of which trigger dysfunctions in our metabolism and immune system.

I believe that the proof of this concept can be seen in the fact that nature has endowed us with many redundant systems in our body to protect us and keep us living. Our DNA is programmed to form us as embryos and to continue repairing the damage that naturally occurs in our cells when we become ill or get hurt, at least for a period of time that is likely as long as 150 years. Our hormonal system determines our growth rate and metabolism and acts to preserve our body in the face of stress and challenge. Our immune system keeps us alive by finding and killing foreign agents that invade our body and eliminating toxins that form in our cells. Our central nervous system, via its neurotransmitters and neuropeptides, controls how all parts of the body communicate with one another, including the circulatory system, the glands, the muscles, and the brain. All these systems are tightly linked to one another, creating a smooth-functioning holistic machine. The hormonal system sparks certain neurotransmitters that then influence our immune system, and the immune system can trigger the hormonal system to go into overdrive, and so on.

Ultimately, what we do to support one bodily system impacts them all. This is why adding ginseng to your diet can have beneficial repercussions throughout your body, leading to a healthier, longer life. Think of your body as you would a car; the more you can facilitate an efficient operation (your metabolism) that runs smoothly, consistently, and with little wear and tear or rust (oxidation), the fewer breakdowns you will have and the less you will need to call in the mechanic (your immune system) to make repairs.

Of course, there is more to ensuring your longevity than taking any one single substance. If you are interested in extending your life span, ginseng should be just one element among many in a well-thought-out and prepared program that includes good nutrition, regular exercise, and a positive, life-sustaining attitude. In fact, almost every study of people who live more than 100 years invariably concludes that these three elements are the key ingredients in extending life span.

In terms of nutrition, a longer life does appear to be correlated to the eating of naturally prepared foods that lack a lot of processed ingredients and are low in saturated fats. As for regular exercise, many enthusiasts today usually recommend an aerobic workout at least three times per week for twenty minutes; however, what seems best for the sake of longevity is actually exercise that takes place outdoors in fresh air and is not inordinately strenuous, such as walking and gardening. Finally, centenarians throughout the world invariably state that they went through life having an optimistic and forward-thinking outlook that kept them going in good times and bad. In the past, many scientists would have discounted such testimony, but today, given what researchers know about the critical roles played by chemicals produced in the brain and nervous system on the immune system and metabolism, there is every reason to endorse this element of a longevity program.

Finally, with increasing research in molecular biology and chemistry today, it is worth listening to the advice of many scientists who suggest that your antiaging program include a variety of nutritional supplements. The main reason for this is that many of us don't eat in the healthiest manner, even if we are diligent about cutting out greasy fast foods and highly processed or refined goods. For most of us, our diet is often weighted with too many calories, too much protein, and too much fat, all of which taxes the body. Also, many people overcook their food, breaking down the nutrients beyond usability. In addition, much of our food is grown in conditions that leech away nutrients or create contaminants, so we do not get all the vitamins, minerals, and trace elements we should.

Nutritional supplements can ensure that you get everything your body needs and, in particular, that you get it in amounts that researchers now believe are more appropriate for increased longevity. Many books suggest daily supplements of the following type and dosage:

▣ multivitamin pill containing at least 100% of the recommended dietary allowance (RDA) of vitamins, minerals, and trace elements, to boost immunity. The pill should also contain at least 400 micrograms of folic acid and no more than 100% of the RDA for iron.

▣ vitamin E supplement containing 100 to 400 IU; vitamin E is considered the best antioxidant.

▣ vitamin C supplement containing 500 to 1,000 milligrams; vitamin C is linked to preventing heart disease and to boosting the immune system, especially against cancer.

▣ beta-carotene supplement containing 10 to 15 milligrams. Beta-carotene works synergistically with vitamins C and E to maintain antioxidant activity in cells.

▣ chromium supplement containing 200 micrograms. Chromium is linked to normalizing blood sugar and improving the ability of insulin to process blood sugar, resulting in a need for less insulin in the body. High levels of insulin can lead to diabetes and heart disease.

▣ selenium supplement containing 50 to 200 micrograms. Selenium is regarded as a potential antiaging agent because it boosts the immune system and protects against heart disease and cancers.

- ▣ calcium supplement of 1,000 milligrams (1,500 for women). Lack of calcium causes bone brittleness, especially in postmenopausal women. Calcium also offsets high sodium levels and thus blocks high blood pressure. Some studies have found that calcium also thwarts the proliferation of cancer-prone cells and fights cholesterol.

- ▣ zinc supplement containing 15 to 30 milligrams. Zinc has been shown to stimulate the thymus gland, which controls the immune system. Insufficient zinc is thought to cause a lowered immune capability to many diseases.

- ▣ magnesium supplement containing 200 to 300 milligrams. Magnesium is linked to preventing heart disease and reducing free radicals.

In addition, many books have other recommendations about other nutritional supplements that you might want to consider based on your lifestyle, family history, and susceptibility to various diseases or illnesses. Whichever way you approach the issue of nutritional supplements, however, ginseng is among the easiest to use, with the most far-reaching results in an antiaging program. Let's look now at how to decide which type of ginseng is right for you.

▣ 7 ▣

Selecting the Right Ginseng for You

The preservation of health is a duty. Few seem conscious that there is such a thing as physical morality.

Herbert Spencer
(1820–1903),
English philosopher

Selecting the right ginseng product for yourself can often seem confusing, given the many varieties of ginseng from around the world and the many commercial brand names you can find in stores. This chapter will explain how to make what is really your first decision: which ginseng, from among the three major types—Asian, Siberian, or American—is best for your body. In the next chapter, we will review how to buy ginseng, including what form of ginseng is best to take—raw root, extract, capsule, tablet, and so on—and what potency or dosage.

The Basis for Your Choice

As you may recall from Chapter 1, there are actually many species of ginseng. Of these, we have mostly limited our discussion in this book to the three main varieties—Asian, American, and Siberian. These three are generally considered throughout the world to be the leading types of ginseng to use, although some devotees from a given part of the world or some manufacturers of a specific brand might endorse only their type of ginseng, claiming it to be far superior to the others. However, such claims are usually motivated by nationalism or the profit incentive.

What truly counts in selecting ginseng is your individual needs! Just as a doctor determines what type of antibiotic to give you based on your ailment and various personal factors such as your age and weight, choosing a ginseng product depends on your physical condition and what you want to use it for. This is because there are significant differences among the three main varieties of ginseng in terms of their strength and efficiency in enhancing your situation. Again, this is because each variety of ginseng has a completely different range of active ingredients, as determined by the actual amount of specific ginsenosides or eleutherosides present. In addition, researchers now recognize that even the ratio of certain active ingredients, such as the ratio of Rg_1 elements to Rb_1 elements in

Panax ginseng, can make a significant difference in the effect and potency of a product.

The following sections explain in detail what most researchers agree are the fundamental characteristics of the three main varieties of ginseng, and which type of person is best suited for each.

Siberian Ginseng—the All-Purpose Antistress Tonic

Although Siberian ginseng is the one primary type of ginseng that is not part of the Panax genus, it is a member of the same family of plants and has many properties in common. Its active ingredients are called eleutherosides, and they are closely related to the ginsenosides found in the other two main species of ginseng. Some people and manufacturing companies refer to Siberian ginseng as *Eleuthero*, because its full botanical name is *Eleutherococcus senticosus*.

Siberian ginseng is considered to be the most adaptogenic of the ginsengs. This means that it is perhaps the best suited to helping people cope with stress, because stress creates unpredictable havoc in the body. If your blood sugar is high, Siberian ginseng will lower it; if your blood sugar is too low, it will raise it. The same moderating influence will be had on other chemicals in your bloodstream under the use of Siberian ginseng.

Like all ginsengs, Siberian enhances your mental and physical performance and causes the adrenal glands to lower the release of the stress hormones that upset the body and negatively affect the immune system. However, it is believed that Siberian ginseng is milder than Asian ginseng and does not stimulate the adrenal glands as dramatically. It can thus be taken by almost anyone for long periods of time without any risk of harmful effects.

As mentioned earlier, Siberian ginseng was heavily researched by Soviet scientists, beginning with Itskovity Brekhman, who tested it on soldiers, athletes, factory and mine workers, and many others. The Soviets used Siberian ginseng for their cosmonauts and their Olympic contenders, especially their weight lifters and runners. In every case, the research indicated good results in improving both mental and physical performance, in reducing sickness (especially in diabetes and heart disease), and in developing a greater tolerance for stress. The results ranged from exceptional gains to modest improvements, but no negative results or toxic effects have ever been reported from the ingestion of Siberian ginseng.

Christopher Hobbs, a noted herbalist and botanist, summarizes the research on Siberian ginseng in this way in his book *The Ginsengs*:

Overall, the studies with human volunteers have helped clarify the broad spectrum of activity for

eleuthero extract. . . . The major physiological effects that have been demonstrated by Russian scientists include a strong antitoxic effect (against environmental toxins), a protective effect against radiation, a normalizing effect against hypothermia, a blood sugar regulating effect, a liver-protective effect, an enhancement of the liver's ability to break down and rid the body of drugs, an increase in the body's ability to resist infection, and adrenal support activity. Most important is eleuthero's positive influence on work capacity and endurance (antifatigue effect), increasing the ability of the cells throughout the body to utilize phosphorus-containing energy molecules and deal with lactic acid and other by-products of metabolism.

In short, Siberian ginseng is perhaps the most all-purpose type of ginseng, suitable for just about any person at any time in life. It can be taken by males and females of any age, beginning in the teens if necessary, but certainly by any adult or senior. Siberian ginseng is perfect for people who are generally healthy but would like to add ginseng to their diet as part of an energizing or rejuvenation/longevity program. It can also be used by people who are suffering from stress and stress-related diseases such as fatigue, chronic fatigue syndrome, diabetes, and heart problems. In either case, Siberian ginseng will produce beneficial effects in strengthening the hormonal system, making healthy individuals feel even healthier day in and day out, or assisting ill people to recover more quickly.

Asian (Chinese or Korean) Ginseng—from "Stimulating" to "Hot"

Asian ginseng is the generic term used to refer to both the Chinese and Korean herb, which are actually the same plant, *Panax ginseng C.A. Meyer*. They are also sometimes simply called Panax ginseng. The difference between Chinese and Korean is simply a question of source, and in the U.S., you can find ginseng from both countries. In fact, many of the products on the commercial market are made from Chinese or Korean ginseng, even if they don't specifically say so.

In general, Asian ginseng is considered to be much more stimulating than Siberian ginseng, and this is attributable to the difference in the chemical composition of its active ingredients. As you may recall, the active ingredients in both species are called saponins; those in Panax ginseng, however, are more specifically termed ginsenosides, whereas those in Siberian are termed eleutherosides. The stimulating nature of Asian ginseng is largely due to the high level of chemicals collectively called Rg1 compounds, which are the most stimulating chemicals among all ginsengs. Asian ginseng is often said to be "hot," because it warms the body by stimulating the hormonal system, which impacts the metabolism, circulatory system, digestion, and many other systems.

In addition, Asian ginseng can be prepared in two different ways, either of which influences how stimulating it becomes. Both Chinese and Korean ginseng can be prepared either by peeling and drying the roots, in which case it is called *white ginseng*, or by steaming them with the skin left on, in which case it is called *red ginseng*. Red ginseng is the "hotter" product, and molecular testing has shown that this method of preparation preserves more of the Rg_1 compounds than the peeling and drying method that creates white ginseng. Many stores carry products labeled Chinese ginseng or Korean ginseng, but the packages do not tell you if the ginseng is red or white. In most cases, the ginseng will be red, because this is easier to prepare and preserves more of the ginsenosides that people want. However, many of the leading brands contain white ginseng.

Asian ginseng is used for the same purposes as Siberian ginseng: to control stress, boost energy, support the immune system, enhance performance, and increase longevity. However, the effects of Asian ginseng on the body are often more dramatic. As a result, Asian ginseng, especially red Chinese or Korean, is sometimes not recommended for children, women, or for anyone who already suffers from a high-speed metabolism, such as those individuals whom we call Type A personalities. For some people, red Asian ginseng may be too stimulating and make them feel nervous and uncomfortable. Some women also experience a change in their normal menstrual cycle when taking red ginseng.

Red ginseng has traditionally been recommended for people who are in need of significant rejuvenation, such as those seriously weakened by fatigue, and for elderly people whose hormonal systems are no longer functioning very well because of age, poor diet, or illness. Traditional Chinese herbal medicine prescribes red ginseng for elders and for people with illnesses that cause sluggishness, lack of motivation, a slow metabolism, and poor circulation.

In my practice, I generally don't recommend Chinese or Korean ginseng to people under the age of forty who are fairly healthy. I usually suggest it for people over forty years old who may be just starting to take ginseng. For such people, it can sometimes be useful to begin with a few months of Korean ginseng before switching to Siberian for the long term. I may also suggest Asian ginseng for people who participate in a lot of intensive sports and thus experience significant depletion of energy in the body. Some athletes combine Asian ginseng with Siberian; Eric Harr takes one capsule of each daily.

American Ginseng

American ginseng is derived from the same Panax genus of plants as Asian ginseng, and so it is very closely related in its ginsenosides. As you may recall, its botanical name is *Panax quinquefolius*, meaning "five-leafed."

Despite its lineage, American ginseng has been determined to contain a very high level of Rb1 ginsenosides, and so the ratio of Rb1 to Rg1 is quite different than that found in Asian ginseng. Because the Rb1 ginsenosides depress rather than stimulate the central nervous system, American ginseng is therefore known to be more calming and "cooler" than its Asian counterpart. In fact, when American ginseng was first discovered in Canada in the early 1700s, it became a significant export crop to Hong Kong and southern China because many Chinese preferred it over their own ginseng, especially in the summer months when people's body temperature tends to be higher anyway.

One might say that American ginseng falls at the other extreme of Asian ginseng, with Siberian ginseng in between. This suggests that American ginseng is suitable for people who need only a slight energy boost or a great amount of antistress tonic to reduce high levels of stress. Some ginseng experts believe that American ginseng is better for Americans than Asian ginseng because Americans already tend to be overly stimulated from the fast pace of our culture and from a diet that emphasizes caffeine, alcohol, tobacco, sugar, and processed foods.

The Yin and Yang of It All

Understanding how to select and use ginseng may seem to be a picky process in our culture, where foods

Hot

More stimulating (more Yang);
Higher percentage of Rg1 component and less of Rb1 component in ginsenosides

Asian Red

Asian White

Neutral

Works as a strong adaptogen; contains both stimulating and calming components in eleutherosides

Siberian

Cold

More calming (more Yin);
Higher percentage of Rb1 component and less Rg1 component in ginsenosides

American

tend to look and taste alike. But just as you can develop an eye and an appreciation for the different species of edible plants, each with its own taste and texture, you can with time also develop more sensitivity to the differences among ginseng plants. It is really no different than learning to prefer one variety of potato over another, or the taste of one wine over another. With practice, your body can tell the difference.

Given that ginseng has been around for thousands of years, it is therefore little wonder that traditional Chinese medicine makes many profound distinctions about how each type of ginseng feels and works. According to the traditional Chinese philosophy of the world, all the forces of nature are divided into a primordial pair: Yin and Yang. These two forces simultaneously complement and oppose each other; as one increases, the other decreases to fill its place. The goal is to achieve a harmony between them. For health to occur, the Yin and Yang in the body must be balanced. There can be neither too much hot nor too much cold, neither too much moisture, nor too much dryness. In traditional Chinese medicine, the Yang forces are associated with the masculine elements of contraction and density, while the Yin forces are associated with the feminine elements of expansion and space.

In this context, health is associated with an even balance of the Yin and Yang forces, and sickness occurs when these elements are not in harmony. Each "disharmony" (meaning problem or disease, although it does not have to be visible or conscious) is different and reflects an overflow or a deficiency in one force or another. For example, someone with severe fatigue or loss of energy may be suffering from a depleted Yang and need a ginseng to "tonify" it to make it stronger. This person would therefore need red ginseng, which is considered to be Yang. In contrast, someone who is suffering from a fever may be lacking in Yin forces and need a tonic to rebalance the Yin in his or her body. This person would benefit from Asian white or perhaps American ginseng, which are considered more Yin.

In general, traditional Chinese medicine has made these affiliations to the various ginsengs:

- *red*—Yang, warming, energizing, stimulating, works on spleen, heart, and lungs

- *white*—Yin, cooling, calming, softening, nourishing, works on heart, lungs, and kidneys

- *American*—Yin, cooling, calming, softening, nourishing, works on heart, lungs, and kidneys

Traditional Chinese medicine is ultimately very complex, and most Americans are not interested in mastering its intricacies or in learning about thousands of other herbs and how they are needed to interact with ginseng. Consequently, it is not useful to go into all the details here about how to select ginseng according to the precepts of traditional Chinese medicine. In fact, in traditional Chinese medicine, the most meaningful way to help someone decide what type of ginseng to take requires examining the person and performing an evaluation. Obviously, this is not possible right now, as I cannot meet you. However, unless you are seriously ill or pregnant, you can feel comfortable following the general recommendations of this chapter, specifically in regard to the conclusions presented below.

If you are interested in learning more about Chinese medicine and its view of the body's energy systems and how they relate to maintaining your health, you can consult many books available at bookstores or attend workshops and conferences given around the country. It is worthwhile to note that ancient Chinese medicine, like the Ayurvedic medical system of India, has become far more intriguing to the West than ever before, because these systems have long considered the mind/body as one holistic unit. This is a view that Western medicine is now beginning to embrace, ironically because more and more research increasingly verifies the integration of body systems and the link between what we think and how we feel. As with ginseng, it may very well turn out that the fundamental precepts of ancient Chinese herbal medicine are more valid than modern science would have ever imagined.

Considering Your Own Factors

In the end, the choice of ginseng must be left to you. Since each of us is a unique person with our own genetic and medical history, our own lifestyle, and our own body metabolism, your decision must be made in light of all of these issues. In selecting the best ginseng variety for you, consider these seven factors:

1. *The reason you want to use the product*—Is it to gain energy, reduce stress, bolster your immune system, enhance your sex life, or add to your longevity? All ginsengs basically accomplish these same tasks but are progressively stronger from American to Siberian to Chinese or Korean.

2. *Your age*—people under forty may prefer American or Siberian; people over forty may benefit more from Siberian or Korean.

3. *Your profession*—people who perform hard physical or mental labor may prefer Siberian or Korean.

4. *Your habitat*—Because of the differences in the "warming" and "cooling" properties of the three main ginsengs, people who live in cold climates may

prefer Chinese or Korean in the winter months and Siberian in the summer. People who live in warm climates may prefer Siberian in the winter months, American in the summer. In general, American ginseng is not as "hot" as Asian, and many people switch to it in the summer months.

5. Your *activity level*—people who are highly active may need to take Siberian or American to reduce their stress, while people who are seeking greater energy or are heavily involved in athletics may prefer Korean or Siberian.

6. Your *gender*—in general, women prefer the cooler Siberian or American, and men prefer hotter Korean, Chinese, or Siberian.

7. Your *emotional condition*—people who feel depressed usually prefer Korean, Chinese, or Siberian; people who feel in need of calming often prefer American.

It may be useful to try whichever type of ginseng you first select for a few weeks or a month on a trial basis. If, after that time, you do not feel any meaningful physical and/or emotional change, or if you feel uncomfortable with these changes you have experienced, you might want to switch to another type of ginseng. Again, remember that ginseng produces no toxic or harmful effects, so even if you don't like the way one type of ginseng makes you feel, all you need to do is stop taking it. Within a day, you will feel back to normal. In all likelihood though, making the transition from one type of ginseng to another will create no problems.

Once you've surpassed the hurdle of what type of ginseng is best for you, you simply need to know how to buy it. In the next chapter, you will see how you can either prepare ginseng yourself or, the more common option, how you can buy commercially prepared ginseng and feel secure that you are getting a well-made, safe product.

The Consumer's Guide to Purchasing Ginseng

There's only one corner of the universe you can be certain of improving, and that's your own self.

Aldous Huxley
(1894–1963),
British author

There are many ways in which you can get ginseng, ranging from going to a Chinese herbalist in the nearest city's Chinatown district, where you can buy a whole root to make your own teas and tinctures, to purchasing a package of capsules at your local health food store or pharmacy. However, unless you have the knowledge and time to make your own teas and tinctures, it is easier to forgo buying a whole root and instead purchase ginseng in a prepared form such as a capsule, tablet, or liquid produced by a reliable manufacturer.

This chapter therefore emphasizes the easiest method of purchasing ginseng. To be able to do this, you need to understand how to select a prepared ginseng product from among the dozens that are currently sold in health food stores, supermarkets, pharmacies, and discount health supply stores. Let's begin by discussing the five rules of choosing ginseng, which will help you feel confident about what type of product you are purchasing, its potency (strength), and its dosage. At the end of the chapter, you will find some additional material about buying a whole root, in case you would like to try that.

Rule #1—Don't Be Misled by Packaging

The first rule of selecting a ginseng product is that you should not be fooled by the design, colors, or shape of the packaging, however official, professional, or beautiful it looks. Ginseng is now a commodity product just like over-the-counter headache pills, cold medicines, or even breakfast cereals, so savvy marketing executives employ many techniques to get you to look at their packages and conclude that their product is better or of higher quality than any other. What truly counts is what's inside, not whether the box is yellow or green or has a picture of a healthy-looking couple smiling back at you. Furthermore, if there is one marketing ploy to watch out for, it's packaging that offers you a rebate or a two-for-one deal; this almost always means that the product is of lower quality. This is because high-quality ginseng is not dirt cheap; it requires many years of cultivation and usually an expensive extraction process that makes it absolutely impossible for anyone to sell the product for only a few dollars. Ginseng products that are sold at rock-bottom prices are simply of inferior quality and have "no therapeutic value," meaning that there is so little potent ginseng in the product that you will derive practically no benefit from it.

Rule #2—Determine the Potency of the Product

The second rule in selecting ginseng is to read the label and determine the true potency or strength of the product. Many companies use different practices in labeling their product, making it difficult to compare from one product to another the amount of ginseng you are actually getting. Unfortunately, some companies are also deceptive in their labeling and lead you to believe that you are getting more than you really are. The reason for much confusion among consumers is that labeling a ginseng product can be done in many ways, and there is no clear standard that allows you to compare products equally.

In general, ginseng is sold either as a liquid, a tablet, or a capsule. Regardless of which delivery system is used, you need to understand exactly how much and of what quality is the ginseng you are buying, so that you can maximize your purchase and be certain that you have bought a bona fide ginseng product. For the purpose of explaining how you can determine its potency, the following section will refer to capsules so that we can simplify the measurements and work only with dry weights.

One method of preparing ginseng is to grind up an entire dried root and put the powder into a capsule. In this case, you can simply measure out an amount of ginseng into each capsule and label it precisely according to its weight. A capsule that contains 100 mg of ginseng powder obviously contains less than another capsule that contains 250 mg.

However, the problem with this production method is that there is a great deal of variation among ginseng roots in the amount of active ingredients. Some roots are simply of higher quality than others and contain more saponins. As a result, many companies use an extraction process whereby they use many pounds of roots and "extract" a concentrated product that is more uniform. In general, the extraction ratio ranges from 2:1 to 5:1; every company is different. As a result, you will find some packages of ginseng that are prepared from concentrated or extracted root, and you can be certain that you are getting a higher quality product because the density of saponins will be greater. A capsule containing 200 mg of ginseng made from extract is almost certain to be better than two capsules of 100 mg made from straight powdered ginseng.

Unfortunately, some companies do not tell you what their extraction ratio is, making it hard to compare products. One package might contain 250 mg capsules made from a 2:1 extraction while the other package has the same 250 mg capsules, but made from a 5:1 extraction. For this reason, it is better to find a product that provides you with as much information as possible so that you can be absolutely certain how much ginseng you are actually getting for the price.

A few companies abuse this method of measuring and produce ginseng that contains both powders and extract, making it hard to truly compare the potency of their product with others. One company, for example, labels their product on the front of the package to indicate that each capsule contains 750 mg of "ginseng equivalent." But if you turn the package around and read the back label, it indicates that the product contains 350 mg of ginseng powder and 100 mg of ginseng extract at a 4:1 ratio. In other words, this company has calculated the total amount of ginseng you are getting in the following manner:

$$\begin{array}{r} 350 \text{ mg of ginseng powder} \\ +100 \text{ mg at 4:1 ratio} = \underline{400 \text{ mg}} \\ 750 \text{ mg} \end{array}$$

This type of labeling is misleading for two reasons. First, it falsely boosts the sense of quality that you think you are purchasing because the portion of the capsule made from ginseng powder is not as good as the portion made from extract. Second, the front of the package advertises 750 mg and thus makes consumers think that they are getting a better buy than another product that contains 250 mg of extract made at a 4:1 ratio. When you first look at the labels, it obviously appears that 750 mg is more than 250 mg, but in truth, if the second company were to multiply out its extraction ratio of 4:1, it could have labeled its product as containing 1,000 mg of ginseng. In other words, the first company is inflating the amount of ginseng you are really getting compared to the labeling practice of most other companies.

The point of this is, when you read the label of any ginseng product, you should check the following:

a) Is the ginseng made from pure root, or is it extracted? (or does the product contain both pure powder and extract?)

b) Can you tell what the extract ratio was? Does the label indicate the extraction or concentration ratio?

c) Can you truly calculate how many milligrams (mg) of ginseng you are really getting?

The best companies indicate on their labels precisely how much total ginseng you are getting and where it is from. Their labels reveal the origin of the ginseng, the total weight of ginseng in each capsule, and what their extraction ratio is. For example, one well-known European company indicates that their Siberian ginseng capsule is 500 mg derived from 2,500 mg of root—hence a 5:1 extraction ratio. Some companies only partially tell what you need to know. For instance, another well-known European manufacturer produces 100 mg capsules made from extract, but it does not reveal that its extract is 4:1, so you cannot accurately compare its product to any other. The worst companies provide you with no information about where the ginseng came from or how it is made. Many lower-priced brands sold in discount health and beauty product stores don't indicate whether they are Chinese, Korean, American, or Siberian ginseng, nor do they reveal in their labeling whether their capsules are made from powder or extract. All you may know is that the capsules contain 250 mg of ginseng.

Rule #3—Look for Standardized Ginseng

In addition to determining the potency of a product, you should also determine if the product has been "standardized." Standardization is the chemical process that ensures that every measure of ginseng has almost precisely the same amount of actual ginsenosides or eleutherosides in it. The best manufacturers can now control the level of active ingredients in every batch of ginseng to such a degree that they can pinpoint the percentage of the actual saponins in a product. For example, many companies that produce Panax ginseng can guarantee each capsule to contain a specific amount of ginsenosides, usually ranging from 4% to 20%. The same can be done for Siberian ginseng products, guaranteeing a specific percentage of eleutherosides in each capsule. Some companies can even chemically isolate specific proportions of ginsenosides to emphasize one property or another. For example, a Panax ginseng can be standardized to contain as high as 29% of the Rg1 component, which would make that product significantly more stimulating than those products that standardize an across-the-board spectrum of saponins.

You may be wondering if it is better to have a product that has a higher standardization percentage; in other words, is it better to buy a product that is guaranteed to contain 5% ginsenosides or eleutherosides rather than 4%? To the extent that a higher percentage of ginsenosides reflects a higher quality, the answer is yes, it is better to have a product that has a higher amount of ginsenosides. However, since you will mostly find only small variations in the guaranteed analysis—just one or two percentage points—the difference between products is usually negligible. What counts more is the overall potency of the product and whether the product is standardized at any level. That way, you can be sure you are getting a good dosage and a consistent amount of ginsenosides in every pill or capsule you take.

Standardization is just as critical as potency when you evaluate a product. Unfortunately, some ginseng products are made from low-quality ginseng roots that might have been too young or grown in poor soil. As a result, this ginseng can contain very low levels of saponins and trace elements, making the products of little therapeutic value.

Rule #4—When Comparing Price, Compare Apples to Apples

Between the potency of a ginseng product and the standardization of its active ingredients, there is a great deal of leeway in the marketplace for buying either a high-quality ginseng product or one of low value. This means that when you compare the price of two products, you need to determine which product is truly the better value. Just like any other product sold by weight or size, you can end up paying a lot of money or a little money per ounce of ginseng, but you must also take into account the quality of what you are buying.

The best way to determine the value of what you are buying is to compare the price per gram of product. First of all, assume that you want to compare two products that are both extracts made at 4:1 ratios, with a guaranteed standardization of 7%. Here's how you compare them:

- Assume Product A is priced at $18 and gives you 30 capsules of 100 mg each. This means that the entire package contains 3,000 mg of ginseng, which is equal to 3 grams. The price translates to $6 per gram. ($18 ÷ 3 gram = $6 per gram).

- Assume Product B costs $24 and gives you 30 capsules of 600 mg each. This means it contains 18,000 mg, which equals 18 grams. Divide $24 by 18 grams, and your cost per gram is $1.33. ($24 ÷ 18 gram = $1.33 per gram). This product is more cost-effective, although on the surface it appears to cost $6 more than the other product. You get more ginseng per dollar.

You also need to determine the price per month for your usage. For example, some bottles have thirty capsules, but require that you take four per day; thus you would need four bottles of the product to last one month. If each bottle costs eight dollars, that's thirty-two dollars per month. Let's say another product costs twenty-four dollars and supplies you with thirty capsules, but at a higher dosage so that you need only one per day. This product would cost you only twenty-four dollars per month.

Rule #5—Buy Your Ginseng from a Reputable Store

As you can see, it can become quite confusing to shop for ginseng. One package might contain capsules of 250 mg of standardized extract but not tell you the extraction ratio, and another product might contain 100 mg of standardized extract at 4:1, but not tell you the guaranteed standardization percentage of ginsenosides, and so on.

For this reason, your best choice is to buy ginseng from a reputable pharmacy, health food store, or other retail outlet that knows its product and carries the best brands. The leading ginseng companies produce high-quality products that are clearly labeled to indicate their potency, extraction ratio, and standardization percentage. Unfortunately, as the market for herbal supplements has grown in recent years, many companies have started selling ginseng products—especially in discount health and beauty products stores—that are not made from extracts and are not standardized. While these products often cost much less, their value is questionable. In fact, in several studies consumer watchdog groups have randomly purchased ginseng sold in supermarkets, pharmacies, and other stores and analyzed the contents of the package to discover that nearly one-half of the products did not have any significant amount of saponins in them. Buying such products is ultimately a total waste of your money.

In my own practice, I recommend that people shop for their ginseng in health food stores, where the most well-known and best companies are usually represented. These products are almost always of higher quality and better value in terms of dollars per gram. You can also feel more secure that you have purchased a well-manufactured and highly controlled product with a good standardization level of ginsenosides or eleutherosides.

Beware of Pesticides

High-quality products are also usually made with ginseng grown in areas without pesticides, which can leave a chemical residue on the roots. Just as chemicals leech into our foods from soils that have been contaminated, pesticides can remain in ginseng roots and eventually enter your body. For this reason, it helps to verify to the best of your ability that the ginseng you purchase comes from fields that have not been chemically treated.

A Note on Other Forms of Prepared Ginseng

Note also that while this chapter has mostly referred to capsules, prepared ginseng is also available in tablets and liquid extract form. However, be aware that many tablets are simply compressed powder or include a combination of other herbs, such as licorice. Capsules are often better because the ginseng extract is mixed into a base paste (often including beeswax, which was also used by the ancient Chinese) that preserves it and makes it fully digestible.

Ginseng liquid extracts are also available for people who prefer to drink the ginseng, but the quality of these likewise depends on the manufacturer. To make the liquid extract, it is recommended that the manufacturer have used "cold pressing" because heat can destroy the natural enzymes in the ginseng root.

In many stores you can often find ginseng teas, in the form of pieces to be used for brewing and in tea bags to make instant tea. Unfortunately, these teas usually contain very little ginseng and are seldom of therapeutic value. Other than drinking them for the flavor and enjoyment as you would any tea, it is best not to think you are getting your daily allotment of ginseng in this way.

Finally, watch out for ginseng cosmetics, skin creams, and "soft drinks." Ginseng, when contained in these types of products, has no value whatsoever.

Even if it is in the product, its dosage is so small that it cannot have any effect on you. The manufacturers of such products have only added enough ginseng so as to be able to use the name "ginseng" to attract the gullible consumer.

Dosage

The dosage of ginseng you ultimately take is critical to its effectiveness. The traditional dosage of ginseng ranges from three to nine grams of Asian or Siberian per day, or from three grams to five grams of American per day. (If you have high blood pressure or heart trouble, do not follow these dosages; you should consult your physician.)

Unfortunately, most people who take ginseng take too small a dosage, which is therapeutically worthless. The main reason for this is that too many manufacturers of capsules and extracts make their dosages far too small, on the order of 100 or 200 mg, and do not indicate the extraction ratio, which is typically only 2:1, or at best 4:1, anyway. This means that you often get less than one gram of ginseng in such products, and the amount of active ingredients (ginsenosides or eleutherosides) that you ingest is virtually ineffective.

Again, many of today's manufacturers seem to suggest on their labels that you need only small amounts of ginseng, far less than the three grams minimum recommended in traditional Chinese medicine. Many packages of ginseng suggest that you take just one capsule per day containing 100 mg. Even assuming these capsules are extracts prepared at a 4:1 or 5:1 ratio, this means that you would be getting less than a half gram of ginseng per day.

In short, you should realize that a therapeutically valuable dosage for most people is between three and nine grams per day. Depending on what type of ginseng you purchase and how many milligrams are in each capsule, you will need to calculate exactly how many capsules or tablets to take to reach this effective dosage. For example, if you were to purchase a product that contains 600 mg capsules made at a 5:1 ratio, each capsule would effectively give you 3,000 mg of ginseng, hence three grams. This means you would want to take one to two capsules per day if you wanted three to six grams per day. A good way to do this would be to take one capsule in the morning and another in the afternoon.

If you want to follow these traditional dosage recommendations, pay attention to which ginseng product you purchase. If you were using one of the well-known products that consist of 100 mg capsules of extract made at a 4:1 ratio, which yields 400 mg of ginseng per capsule, you would need to take eight capsules to get your three grams per day, or sixteen capsules if you wanted to take six grams per day.

This is why some of the "mass-marketed" ginseng products are actually very expensive compared to the products sold at health food stores, whose dosage levels are usually higher, thus requiring you to take only one or two capsules per day to achieve a therapeutic effect. *Remember: when comparing products, calculate your daily cost in grams, not just by capsule count.*

In my own practice, I follow the traditional Chinese dosage and generally recommend at least three grams per day, and often recommend an even higher dosage of six grams per day. Smaller amounts than this are minimally effective, despite what many companies lead you to believe! Of course, each person must determine his or her own proper dosage. If you are feeling especially tired, are undertaking more sports, or are experiencing more stress, you may wish to begin with the highest dosage I recommend, six to nine grams per day.

Again, ginseng has never been shown to be harmful at high dosages, so there is little need to be concerned about ingesting from three to nine grams per day if that is what you feel you need. In fact, some world-class athletes have taken up to fifteen grams of ginseng per day.

On the other hand, some experts recommend that serious athletes who are involved in competitions do not take the highest dosages recommended, but instead take only one or two grams per day for several months at a time. The reason for this is that athletes often take their body "to the edge" during training and competition, and too much ginseng can produce symptoms of headaches, muscle tension, insomnia, and heat signs. However, a normal dosage of ginseng around one or two grams will suffice.

Note: If you are taking one capsule per day, it is best to take it in the morning with water. Take the capsule twenty minutes before eating so as not to have the digestion of food interfere with your body's proper absorbtion of the saponins. If you are taking more than one capsule per day, split your dosage between morning and afternoon, taking two or three grams in the morning, and another three grams in the late afternoon. In general, don't take ginseng late in the day or in the evening, as it may stimulate your body too much and interfere with your sleep.

How Long Should You Take Ginseng?

The first aspect of answering this question is to recognize that tonic herbs take time to work. While you may experience results within a few days of starting to take ginseng, it is best to give it at least two weeks to two months to truly produce consistent effects in stress reduction, increased energy and endurance, and a feeling of well-being. Remember that ginseng is a natural product derived from an herb, not a chemical synthesized in a pharmaceutical laboratory. As mentioned earlier, research has shown that your body absorbs the nutrients from natural products much more fully than from synthesized drugs. Nevertheless, you need to allow herbal products to reach a saturation level in your body before you can experience a true therapeutic effect.

The second part of this question has to do with the length of time you should continue taking ginseng. The traditional Chinese wisdom is that, provided there are no harmful effects, you can take ginseng continuously for years. I am generally not adverse to this approach. My father has taken ginseng continuously for twenty years; he is now in his eighties and still has an active life, living both in Europe and the United States. He functions at a much younger biological age than most eighty-year-old men.

However, many other experts suggest that you take ginseng for two or three months at a time, then halt your usage for one month and start again. When you start again, you may want to see if another variety of ginseng has different beneficial effects on you, or if you live in a climate that has a change of seasons, you may want to change to a "cooler" or "warmer" ginseng as discussed in the previous chapter. I have seen this seasonal method be effective for many people; it seems that after the initial period of two or three months, the body reaches a plateau. Then, when you restart a new period, the body renews itself and moves to a new plateau, where you experience another increase in energy, stamina, and performance.

Becoming an Herbalist—Buying Whole Roots

If you have access to an herbal dealer, such as in the Chinatown area of the nearest city, you might consider purchasing a whole root and experimenting with making your own ginseng tea, decoctions, and tinctures. If you decide to purchase a whole root, be sure to find a reputable dealer who can help you learn to judge the age of the root (a high-quality root must be at least five to six years old, perhaps even eight) and how to assess how the root was preserved to ensure its saponin content. If you misjudge or are misinformed, you can end up with a root that is too young—or perhaps not even ginseng. There are, unfortunately, many scams in the ginseng root market, such as selling a low-grade root as if it were a more expensive high-grade one. Some sellers will even go so far as to glue the root hairs from an expensive Chinese root onto the stock of an American root and sell it as if it were an expensive and venerable Chinese root. As the saying goes when you are in any marketplace you do not know, *caveat emptor*—buyer beware!

To assess the age of a root, find one with the neck (the stalk above the crown) still on it, since this is how you can tell its age. A greater number of fine lines forming rings around the crown usually indicates an older root.

Roots are also graded according to quality. Whether you buy a ginseng root from a mail-order company or in a store, you will likely see a number along with the name. This number indicates the size of the root in terms of how many roots it takes to make a "catty" (1.3 pounds). A lower number means a more valuable root, since older roots are larger and fewer larger roots are needed to make a catty. (The most valuable roots are five to seven years old.) Thus, a root numbered "25" is more valuable than a root numbered "45." There is also another grading system that goes simply from #1 to #3, with #1 being the better root. This system is commonly used in Asia and is reliable.

Remember, you can find many types of roots, from wild to woods-grown to cultivated. In general, Chinese wild roots are almost impossible to find in the American market, since most of them have already been picked and there are far fewer naturally wild areas left in China. For the most part, you will find the following types of roots at Chinese herbal shops:

- ▣ "semi-wild" Yi sun Chinese roots that have been grown in natural forested areas

◙ cultivated Shiu chu or Kirin roots, grown on farms

◙ woods-grown American roots (attention: some may be treated with pesticides)

◙ cultivated American roots, grown on farms in the United States and Canada

In addition, several other species of ginseng may be found in herbal shops, including:

◙ *Brazilian ginseng*, which has some of the same effects as Asian ginseng and may have adaptogenic properties, although it is not a member of the Panax family.

◙ *Indian ginseng*, one the most important plants in Ayurvedic medicine in India, used to treat fatigue, general weakness, impotence, and infertility. This herb is not a member of the Panax family, and is presumed to contain other chemicals than the ginsenosides found in Chinese and Korean ginseng.

◙ *American red ginseng*, which is American ginseng from Michigan or Wisconsin that has been steamed like red Chinese or Korean ginseng. This process makes the American ginseng much "hotter," and thus is somewhat of an anomaly, given that most people prefer American ginseng because it is cooler and more calming than Chinese and Korean.

▣ *American red desert ginseng*, which is grown in the Southwest and is actually the plant known as caniagre (*Rumex hymenosepalus*). This plant is not related to ginseng at all and is considered a fraud by most knowledgeable experts; this ginseng has no adaptogenic properties.

▣ *Alaskan ginseng*, which is actually the plant Devil's Club (*Oplopanax horridum*). This plant is, like Siberian ginseng, a member of the Araliaceae family, and was used by some Native American tribes to lower blood sugar levels in diabetics. It may have adaptogenic properties similar to Siberian ginseng, but further research is needed.

Making Your Own Ginseng Brews

Here are a few recipes to try if you would like to prepare your own ginseng brew:

Ginseng Tea

Cut the ginseng root into slices and place it in hot water in a nonmetal pot. (To avoid contaminating the brew with metal residues that can eliminate the antioxidizing properties of ginseng, it is best to use an enamel, ceramic, or glass pot, or, as the Chinese do, a pure silver pot.) Cover a slice of root weighing about a quarter ounce with water and bring to a near boil for forty-five minutes to one hour. That is your tea. If you want, you can also repeat the process with another round of water to make a "double decoction," since the roots are expensive and may be worth boiling twice. Keep the water from either brew for up to four days in your refrigerator, making cups of tea from it as you desire. Some people add ginger slices to flavor the tea.

Some experts recommend that you make seven ounces of tea from each quarter ounce of ginseng. Then drink one ounce of tea each day. If you make twenty-eight ounces of tea from each quarter ounce of ginseng root, then drink four ounces each day. In other words, follow the ratio of a quarter ounce of raw root to seven ounces of liquid, and drink the appropriate multiple of one ounce of liquid per day.

Ginseng Tincture

Take one ounce or so of sliced ginseng root and place it into a quart of liquor, such as vodka. Recap the bottle tightly and age it for three months. The resulting "tincture" is what you can use for your daily usage, about one ounce at a time.

Another recipe is to grind up the root (after at least one hour of soaking) in a blender and make a "smoothie," using vodka. Let the solids settle down in the mixture; make sure you have about two inches of eighty-proof vodka covering the solids at the bottom to prevent them from rising to the surface and fermenting in the air. Shake the blend every day for two weeks and then strain it through a cheesecloth or linen cloth. Filter this liquid through a paper coffee filter if you want to clarify it. Drink a few half-teaspoonfuls per day of this tincture.

Chewing the Raw Root

Some people simply like the flavor of ginseng when chewed raw. Let a small sliver of root sit in your mouth to soften for a while. Then slowly chew it into small pieces, and swallow them little by little.

These alternative methods of taking ginseng are fun and worth exploring if you want to experience some of the ritual and tradition behind ginseng. However, I would not generally use them as your primary way to get a good dosage of ginseng into your body on a regular basis. For this, I highly recommend the purchase of capsules that have been made from extract and are standardized.

Enjoying Your Newfound Energy and Vitality

Ginseng can be a valuable nutritional supplement for almost anyone. As you have seen throughout this book, ginseng offers many beneficial effects, including:

- boosting your ability to cope with stress

- reducing stress hormones that block the immune system

- enhancing your metabolism and oxygen absorption

- improving the function of the liver

- increasing your mental acuity and physical endurance

- preventing the build-up of many chemicals in the blood, including the bad LDL cholesterol

- reducing the risk of heart disease, diabetes, certain cancers, and many other age- and stress-related illnesses

When you put it all together, there is truly no other herb that has yet been discovered on the face of this planet that offers as many potent and life-giving health benefits as ginseng. What thousands of years of ancient Chinese medicine have shown us based on a simpler system of medicine and a much less complete understanding of physiology and chemistry, we now know to be largely true. Clearly, more experimentation and research is needed in specific areas to even better understand the effects and properties of ginseng. But you can feel confident that by adding ginseng to your diet you will improve your health and well-being in ways you never imagined.

So give ginseng a try. Get the ginseng edge in your life today.

Bibliography

Books

Bensky, Dan, and Gamble, Andrew. *Chinese Herbal Medicine: Materia Medica*. Seattle: Eastland Press, 1986.

Bergner, Paul. *The Healing Power of Ginseng & the Tonic Herbs*. Rocklin, CA: Prima Publishing, 1996.

Brekhman, I. I. *Man and Biologically Active Substances: The Effect of Drugs, Diet, and Pollution on Health*. New York: Pergamon Press, 1980.

Carper, Jean. *Stop Aging Now!* New York: Harper-Collins, 1995.

Dixon, Pamela. *Ginseng.* London: Duckworth, 1976.

Donadieu, Yves. *Le Ginseng: Therapeutique Naturelle.* Paris, France: Librairie Maloine, 1985.

Donsbach, Kurt W. *Ginseng.* Rosarito Beach, Baja, CA: Wholistic Publications, 1981.

Edde, Gerard. *Ginseng et plantes toniques.* Paris, France: Editions Dangles, 1995.

Foster, Steven. *American Ginseng.* American Botanical Council, 1991.

Foster, Steven. *Siberian Ginseng.* American Botanical Council, 1991.

Foster, Steven. *Asian Ginseng.* American Botanical Council, 1991.

Fulder, Steven. *Ginseng and Other Chinese Herbs for Vitality.* Rochester, VT: Healing Arts Press, 1980.

Fulder, Steven. *An End to Aging: Remedies for Life Extension.* New York: Destiny Books, 1983.

Fulder, Steven. Ginseng: *The Magical Herb of the East.* London: Thorsons, 1988.

Halstead, Bruce W., and Hood, Loretta L. *Eleuthero-coccus Senticosus: Siberian Ginseng: An Introduction to the Concept of Adaptogenic Medicine.* Long Beach, CA: Oriental Healing Arts Institute, 1984.

Hammer, Daniel, M.D., and Burr, Barbara. *Peak Energy.* New York: St. Martins, 1988.

Harriman, Sarah. *The Book of Ginseng.* New York: Pyramid Publications (Harcourt), 1976.

Hayflick, Leonard. *How and Why We Age.* New York: Ballantine Books, 1994.

Hobbs, Christopher. *The Ginsengs: A User's Guide.* Santa Cruz, CA: Botanica Press, 1996.

Kamen, Betty. *Siberian Ginseng: Up-to-Date Research on the Fabled Tonic Herb.* New Canaan, CT: Keats Publishing, Inc., 1988.

Kisaki, Kuniyoshi, M.D. *Miracle Korean Ginseng.* Seoul: Korean Ginseng Research Institute, 1980.

Klatz, Ronald, M.D., and Goldman, Robert, M.D. *Stopping the Clock.* New Canaan, CT: Keats Publishing, Inc., 1988.

Lee, Florence C. *Facts About Ginseng: The Elixir of Life.* Elizabeth, New Jersey: Hollym, 1992.

Mowrey, Daniel B. *Herbal Tonics*. New Canaan, CT: Keats Publishing, Inc., 1990.

Mowrey, Daniel B. *Next Generation Herbal Medicine*, Second Edition. New Canaan, CT: Keats Publishing, Inc., 1996.

Murray, Michael T., N.D., *Chronic Fatigue Syndrome*. Rocklin, CA: Prima Publishing, 1994.

Murray, Michael T., N.D., *Stress, Anxiety, and Insomnia*. Rocklin, CA: Prima Publishing, 1995.

Persons, Scott W. *American Ginseng: Green Gold*. Asheville, NC: Bright Mountain Books, 1986.

Selye, Hans. *Stress Without Distress*. Philadelphia: J. B. Lippincott Company, 1974.

Whitaker, Julian, M.D. *Dr. Whitaker's Guide to Natural Healing*. Rocklin, CA: Prima, 1995.

Yeung, Him-che. *Handbook of Chinese Herbs and Formulas*. Los Angeles: Institute of Chinese Medicine, 1985.

Articles

The following articles are all scholarly publications from researchers, doctors, or professors in academic facilities or pharmaceutical companies. The articles are listed by author, name of article, publisher information, and date.

Dorling, Eberhard. "Action of a Preparation Containing a Standardized Ginseng Extract on Physical and Mental Performance." *Arztliche Praxis*, 41, 50: 1867–1869, (1989).

Chinna, Christian. "Panax Ginseng—a Survey." *Oesterreichische Apotheker-Zeitung*, 37, 51/52: 1022–1027, (1983).

Forgo, I., M.D. "The Effect of Different Ginsenoside Concentrations on Physical Work Capacity." *Notabene Medici*, 12, 9: 721–727, (1982).

Forgo, I., M.D. "Effect of Drugs on Physical Performance and Hormone System of Sportsmen." Therapeutic Research Dept. of the Medical University Policlinic, Basel, Switzerland, (1983).

Forgo, I., M.D. "Effect of Standardized Ginseng Extract on General Well-Being, Reaction Capacity, Pulmonary Function, and Gonadal Hormones." *Medizinische Welt*, 32, 19: 751–756, (1981).

Forgo, I., M.D. "The Duration of Effect of the Standardized Ginseng Extract G115 in Healthy Competitive Athletes." *Notabene Medici*, 15, 9: 636–640, (1985).

Forgo, I., M.D., and Kirchdorfer, A.M., M.D. "On the Question of Influencing the Performance of Top Sportsmen by Means of Biologically Active Substances." Medical Science Department of the Interhealth Foundation, Liechtenstein, (1981).

Goode, R. C., Chatha, D., Baker, J., Mertens, T., and Mertens, R. "The Effects of Ginseng on Physical Performance in Human Subjects." Department of Physiology, Faculty of Medicine, University of Toronto, Ontario, (1995).

Hugonot, R., Hugonot, L., and Israel, L. "Clinical Double-Blind Study of Geriatric Pharmaton Against Placebo on 98 Patients, Aged 50 and More, During 60 Days." Centre Hospitalier Regionale et Universitaire de Grenoble, France, (1981).

Mulz, D. and Degenring, F. "Doping Control After a 14-Day Treatment." Pharmaton SA, Lugano, Switzerland, Pharmazeutische Rundshau 11: 22, (1989).

Neri, M., Andermarcher, E., Pradelli, J., and Salvioli, J. "Influence of a Double-Blind Pharmacological Trial on Two Domains of Well-Being in Subjects with Age Associated Memory Impairment." Archives of Gerontology and Geriatrics, 21; 241–252, (1995).

Owen, R. T., M.D. "Ginseng: A Pharmacological Profile." *Drugs of Today*, 17, 8: 343–351, (1981).

Pieralisi, Giuliana, Ripari, P., and Vecchiet, L. "Effects of a Standardized Ginseng Extract Combined with Dimethylaminoethanol Bitartrate, Vitamins, Minerals, and Trace Elements on Physical Performance During Exercise." *Clinical Therapeutics*, 13, 3, (1991).

Quiroga, Hector, M.D., and Imbriano, A. "The Effect of Panax Ginseng Extract on Cerebrovascular Deficits." *Orientacion Medica*, 28, 1208: 86–87, (1979).

Ragusin, Jorge E. "Clinical Trial of a New Product for the Prevention and Treatment of Symptoms Associated with Senility." Department of Geriatrics, Central Military Hospital, Buenos Aires, Argentina, (1980).

Tesch, Per A., Johansson, H., and Kaiser, P. "The Effect of Ginseng, Vitamins, and Minerals on the Physical Work Capacity in Middle-Aged Men." *Lakartidningen*, 84, 51: 4326–4328, (1987).

Ussher, Jane M. "The Relationship Between Health Related Quality of Life and Dietary Supplementation in British Middle Managers: A Double-Blind

Placebo Controlled Study." *Psychology and Health*, 10: 97–111, (1995).

Wiklund, Ingela, Karlberg, J., and Lund, B. "A Double-Blind Comparison of the Effect on Quality of Life of a Combination of Vital Substances Including Standardized Ginseng G115 and Placebo." *Therapeutic Research*, 55, 1, (1994).

Index

ACTH (adrenocorticotropic hormone), 47, 59–60, 130
Adaptation energy, 52–53
Adaptogens, 11, 62
  criteria, 28–29
  medical importance of, 36–39
Adrenal glands, 47, 49, 58–59, 129–30
Adrenaline (epinephrine), 47–50, 129–30
Aerobic metabolism, 83
Aging, 152–54. *See also* Longevity
  biological theories
    genetic control, 163–64, 167–68
    neuroendocrine, 160–63, 167
  random theories, 154–56
    free radical, 158–60, 165–67
    immune system, 160, 166
    wear and tear, 156–58, 164–65
Alarm phase, of GAS model, 47–48

Alaskan ginseng, 214
Alcohol, 111–13
Allopathic doctors, 27
Alternative medicine, 27
American ginseng (*Panax quinquefolius*), 5–6, 33, 36
  history of, 25–26
  properties of, 185–86
  roots, 213
  saponins in, 32
American red desert ginseng, 214
American red ginseng, 213
Anabolic steroids, 85–86
Anabolism, 83–84
Anaerobic metabolism, 83
Anemia, 139–40
Antioxidants, 159
Aphrodisiacs
  chemistry of, 105–8
  defined, 105

foods and herbs as, 106–8
ginseng and, 23–24, 108–11
myth versus fact, 97–101
Araliaceae (ginseng). *See* Ginseng
(*Araliaceae*)
Asian ginseng (*Panax ginseng* C. A.
Meyer), 5, 33, 36, 114
Korean type of, 5, 114
red, 183–84, 186
saponins in, 32
standardization of, 200
uses for, 182–84
white, 183, 186
Asparagus, as aphrodisiac, 106–7
Astrology, 23
Athletics, 76–78
ATP (adenosine triphosphate), 61, 84
ATPase, 61, 84
Attitudes, 172–73
Autoimmune diseases, 125–26
Automatic nervous system, 102
Ayurvedic medicine, 189

B cells, 50
Bank of adaptation energy, 52
Benzel, R., 92–93
Beta-carotene, 174
Beta-sitosterol, 35
Boone, D., 26
Brazilian ginseng, 213
Brekhman, I. I., 28–31, 72, 135, 168, 180
Bruises, 136

Calcium, 119, 174
Cancer treatments, 145–47
Castor beans, 18
Catabolism, 83–85
Catty, 212
Cell death, 163–64
CFS (chronic fatigue syndrome),
125–26, 140–42
Chi, 20–21
China, 19–20
Chinese ginseng. *See* Asian ginseng
Chinese medicine
ginseng and, 19–20, 187–89
medicinal herb classifications,
21–22
tenets of, 22

Chocolate, as aphrodisiac, 107
Cholesterol, 137, 143
Choline, 89, 117
Chromium, 120, 174
Chronic fatigue syndrome. *See* CFS
(chronic fatigue syndrome)
Cinchona bark, 18
Colds, 135–36
Cortisone, 130
Cosmetics, ginseng, 205–6
Cousins, N., 38
Crocker, B., 93–94

Damiana, 108
Death, 52
Depression, 148–49
Devil's Club (Oplopanax horridum),
214
DHEA (dehydroepiandrosterone),
161–62
Diabetes, 137–39
Diet. *See also* Nutrition
and sexual health, 115–22
stress, 42
Digestive ailments, 136–37
Digitalis, 18
Diseases, 46–53, 124–27
DNA (deoxyribonucleic acid),
163–64
Dopamine, 103
Doping substances, 86
Dosages, 206–9

Eleutherococcus senticosus.
See Siberian ginseng
(*Eleutherococcus*
senticosus)
Eleutherosides, 11, 32, 34–35, 182
Endocrine system, 103, 127–32, 136
Endorphins, 128, 133–34
Ephedra sinica, 9–10
Epinephrine (adrenaline), 47–50,
129–30
Epstein-Barr virus, 141
Estrogen, 103
Exercise, 37, 42, 172
Exhaustion phase, of GAS model,
50–53, 141
Extraction ratios, 196–97

Fatigue, 140–42
Fertility, 113–14
Fight or flight phase, of GAS model,
    47–48
Fight or flight syndrome, 100
Flavonoids, 35
Flu, 135–36
Foods, as aphrodisiacs, 106–7
Foxglove, 18
Free radical theory of aging, 158–60,
    165–66
Fulder, S., 55, 59, 63–64

General Adaptation Syndrome (GAS)
    defined, 46–47
    phases
            alarm, 47–48
            exhaustion, 50–53
            resistance, 48–50
Generalized fatigue, 140–42
Generalized illnesses, 135–36
Genetic control theory of aging,
    163–64, 167–68
Gilmond, D., 92
Gilmond, J., 92
Ginseng (Araliaceae), 1–2, 5. See also
    Alaskan ginseng; American
    ginseng; Asian ginseng; Indian
    ginseng; Red ginseng; Siberian
    ginseng; White ginseng
    active ingredients in, 31–36
    adaptive properties of, 54–57
    adaptogen properties of, 28–30,
        34–35
    as adaptogen/antistress agent, 62–66
    aging theories and, 164–68
    American use of, 26–28
    anatomy, 4–5
    as antidote to alcohol, 111–13
    as aphrodisiac, 23–24, 108–11
    beneficial effects, 90–94, 216–17
    capsules, 8–9
    chemical properties, 35–36, 57–60
    as Chinese herbal medicine, 19–22
    Chinese lore and, 23–24
    compounds in, 35–36
    cultivation, 6–7
    derivation, 4
    determining potency, 195–99

    dosages, 206–9
    European use of, 25
    factors for selecting, 190–92
    grading, 23
    immune systems and, 132–35
    improving mental performance
        with, 86–90
    length for taking, 209–11
    metabolism and, 60–62
    packaging, 194–95
    physical performance and,
        72–76
    preparation, 7–9
    pricing, 201–3
    purchasing, 203–6
    safety of, 9–11
    selecting, 178–79
    sex and, 108–11, 114–15
    species, 213–14
    sports performance and, 76–78
    standardization, 199–201
    stress reduction and, 53–57, 67–68
    stress–disease connection and,
        124–27
    varieties, 3–7
Ginsenosides, 11, 32, 143, 182
Glucocorticoid hormones, 49, 130

Harr, E., 78–81, 136, 184
Harsh environments, 54–55
Healing process, 136
Heart disease, 142–43
Herbs, 3–4
    as aphrodisiacs, 106–8
    Chinese classifications, 21–22
    Chinese medicine and, 19–22
    early civilizations and, 17–18
High blood pressure, 137, 143
HIV patients, 147
Hobbs, C., 180
Homeostasis, 43
Honey, as aphrodisiac, 107
Hydrocortisone, 49, 130
Hypertension, 137
Hypothalamus, 59–60
    aging and, 160–61

Immune system theory of aging, 160,
    166

Immune systems, 132–35
India, 24
Indian ginseng, 213
Inflammations, 136
Insomnia, 148–49
Insulin, 137–38
Interferon, 134–35, 141–42
Iodine, 18, 121

Japan, 24
Jarteux, Father, 25

Ketone bodies, 138
Kirin ginseng roots, 213
Korea, 24
Korean ginseng. See Asian ginseng

Labels, ginseng, 197–99
Lao-tzu, 20
Laughter, 37
Lazarev, N. V., 28–31
Lecithin, 117
Liquid extracts, ginseng, 205
Liver, role of, in stress reduction, 61
Longevity. See also Aging
    factors, 170–72
    ginseng's role in increasing, 168–70
    nutrition and, 172–75
Love Potions: A Guide to Aphrodisiacs
    and Sexual Pleasures (Watson),
    109–10, 118
Love-making, 96–97

Ma huang, 9–10
Magnesium, 120, 175
Manganese, 121
Menopause, 143
Mental performance, 55, 71, 86–90
Metabolism, 60–62, 83
Meyer, C. A., 5
Minerals, 119–22
Mitochondria, 157–58
Mood problems, 148–49
Morrow, D., 144
Mowrey, D. R., 34
Multivitamins, 174

Native Americans, 25
Negative feedback loop, 49

Neuroendocrine theory of aging,
    160–63, 167
Neuropeptides, 103
Neurotransmitters, 103–4
Niacin (B-3), 116
NK (natural killer) cells, 50, 141–42
Nonspecific stress responses, 62
Noradrenaline (norepinephrine),
    129–30
Normal aging, 153
Nutrition, 172–75. See also Diet
Nutritional supplements, 173–75

Oxidation, 159
Oxytocin, 107
Oysters, as aphrodisiac, 110

Panax ginseng C. A. Meyer. See Asian
    ginseng (Panax ginseng C. A.
    Meyer)
Panax quinquefolius. See American
    ginseng (Panax quinquefolius)
Pancrease, 129
Pantothenic acid (B-5), 121
Parathyroids, 129
Pathologic aging, 153
Pesticides, 204
Phenolic compounds, 35
Phenylalanine, 111
Physical labor, 54–55
Physical performance, 71, 72–76
Pituitary gland, 59–60, 128
Placebo effect, 99
Polysaccharides, 35
Pregnancy, 113–14
Prepared ginseng, 205–7
Preventative medicine, 28
Progesterone, 103

Quinine, 18

Radiation treatments, 145–47
Rb1 group of saponins, 32–33
Red ginseng, 7–8, 114, 183, 184
Relaxation techniques, 42
Resistance phase, 48–50
Rg1 group of saponins, 32–33
Riboflavin (B-2), 116
Rogaine, 99–100

Roots, ginseng
  assessing age of, 212
  brewing, 214–16
  buying, 211
  eating raw, 216
  grading, 212
  species, 213–14
  types, 212–13

Saponins, 31–32, 58, 64, 182
Saunas, 37
Seaweed, 18
Selenium, 120, 174
Selye, H., 43–46, 51, 53, 62
Serotonin, 103
Sex, 95–97
  bodily systems functions required
    for, 102–4
  diet and, 115–22
  ginseng and, 108–11, 114–15
  phases of, 101
Shiu chu ginseng roots, 213
Siberian ginseng (Eleutherococcus
    senticosus), 6, 30, 34–35, 36, 186
  properties of, 179–82
  saponins in, 32
  standardization of, 200
Soft drinks, ginseng, 205–7
Sports performance, 76–78
Stamina, 55–56
Standardized ginseng, 199–201
Steroids, 64
  anabolic, 85–86
Stress
  disease and, 46–53
  effects, 42
  principles, 44–46
  reducing, 67–68
  scientific view of, 43–46
  traditional approaches for
    eliminating, 42

Stress reduction
  ginseng and, 53–57
  role of liver in, 61
Stress–disease connection, 124–27
Stressors, 43
Surgery, 144–45

Tablets, ginseng, 205
Teas, ginseng, 8, 205, 214–15
Testosterone, 103
Thiamin (B-1), 116
Thymus, 129
Thyroid, 128
Tinctures, 8, 215–16
Trace minerals, 35
Triterpenoids, 64
Type I diabetes, 138
Type II diabetes, 138–39

Vietnam, 24
VIP (vasoactive intestinal peptide), 103
Vitamin B-5 (Pantothenic acid), 117
Vitamin B-1 (Thiamin), 116
Vitamin B-3 (Niacin), 116
Vitamin B-12, 117
Vitamin B-2 (Riboflavin), 116
Vitamin C, 118, 174
Vitamin E, 119, 174
Vitamins, 115–18

Watson, C., 105–6, 114
Wear and tear theory of aging, 156–58,
    164–65
Western medicine, 189
White ginseng, 7, 183

Yi sun Chinese ginseng roots, 212
Yin and Yang, 21, 186–90
Yohimbine, 107

Zinc, 119, 175

▣ About the Author ▣

Jacques MoraMarco, O.M.D., is a licensed acupuncturist in California with more than twenty years of experience in Eastern medical practice. Born in Switzerland, he has studied throughout the United States, Europe, and the Orient, including the École Européen d'Acupuncture in Paris, France. He has a bachelor's degree in biology from Loyola University (Los Angeles), and a doctorate in Oriental medicine from the California Acupuncture College (now known as The Pacific College of Oriental Medicine), where his studies included acupuncture, herbology, tai chi, and Tui-na (Chinese medicinal massage). Dr. MoraMarco is a pioneer in Oriental medicine in the United States, receiving in 1977 the first board-certified acupuncture license granted in the state of California.

Through his studies, Dr. MoraMarco became fascinated with Chines herbology, particularly ginseng—the leading herb in Chinese pharmacopoeia. His interest led him to tour the world's leading research facilities to examine ginseng production, biochemical analysis, and manufacture. His work in this field has made him a recognized expert in ginseng and Chinese herbology; he lectures throughout the world at symposiums and colleges of Oriental medicine.

Dr. MoraMarco resides in Palm Springs, California, where he maintains a private practice in Oriental medicine and teaches at the College of the Desert.